Paediatric and Neonatal Critical Care Transport

Paediatric and Neonatal Critical Care Transport

Edited by

Peter Barry
Consultant Paediatric Intensivist, Children's Intensive Care Service,
University Hospitals of Leicester and Honorary Senior Lecturer,
University of Leicester

Andrew Leslie
Neonatal Transport Coordinator/Advanced Neonatal Nurse Practitioner,
Nottingham Neonatal Service, City & University Hospitals, Nottingham

© BMJ Publishing Group 2003
BMJ Books is an imprint of the BMJ Publishing Group

First published in 2003
3   2006
by BMJ Books, BMA House, Tavistock Square,
London WC1H 9JR

British Library Cataloguing in Publication Data
A catalogue record for this book is available from the British Library
ISBN 13: 978-0-7279-1770-6
ISBN 10: 0-7279-1770-6

Typeset by SIVA Math Setters, Chennai, India

Contents

Contributors

Peter Barry
Consultant Paediatric Intensivist, Children's Intensive Care Service, University Hospitals of Leicester and Honorary Senior Lecturer, University of Leicester

Sandie Bohin
Consultant Neonatologist, University Hospitals of Leicester

David Field
Professor of Neonatal Medicine, University of Leicester, Honorary Consultant Neonatologist, University Hospitals of Leicester

Julie Hall
Neonatal Transport Coordinator, University Hospitals of Leicester

Taj Hassan
Consultant in Emergency Medicine, The General Infirmary at Leeds, Leeds Teaching Hospitals Trust

Carmel Hunt
Paediatric Retrieval Coordinator, Children's Intensive Care Service, University Hospitals of Leicester

Andrew Leslie
Neonatal Transport Coordinator/Advanced Neonatal Nurse Practitioner, Nottingham Neonatal Service, City and University Hospitals, Nottingham

David Luyt
Consultant Paediatric Intensivist, Paediatric Intensive Care Service, University Hospitals of Leicester

Andrew MacIntyre
Consultant Paediatric Intensivist, Royal Hospital for Sick Children, Glasgow

Sanjiv Nichani
Consultant Paediatric Intensivist, Paediatric Intensive Care Service, University Hospitals of Leicester

Giles Peek
Honorary Lecturer in Cardiothoracic Surgery and ECMO, University of Leicester

Moira Robinson
Senior Medical Technician, Paediatric Intensive Care Service, University Hospitals of Leicester

David Rowney
Consultant in Paediatric Anaesthesia and Intensive Care, Royal Hospital for Sick Children, Edinburgh

David Vickery
Consultant in Emergency Medicine, Gloucestershire Royal Hospital

Acknowledgements

Many people offered helpful opinions, advice and criticism as we wrote this manual. We would like to acknowledge the important contributions made by all the people, past and present, who have taught on the Paediatric and Infant Critical Care Transport course in Leicester. The course grew with the experience and contributions of those people, and this book grew from the course. *Paediatric and Neonatal Critical Care Transport* is now the coursebook for NEOSTAR, a course run by the Advanced Life Support Group.

Our thanks go to Jackie Howarth, who currently administers the transport course, and to Caroline Clay, for her secretarial help.

Our thanks also to the transport teams in Leicester and Nottingham and to Merran Thomson, David Thomas, Rose Kent, Kate Wilson, Tracy Earley, Jenny Burgess, Mary Merriman, Lynda Raphael, Charlotte Huddy, Ian Buck Barrett, Martin Earley, Amanda Bowman, Colin Read, Manjeet Riyat and Ashish Chickermane.

The manual was expertly guided to fruition by Mary Banks, Christina Karaviotis and the team at BMJ Books. SIVA Math Setters took our crude sketches and turned them into the attractive illustrations seen in this manual.

Every effort has been made to ensure the accuracy of the data, particularly drug doses, in this manual, but it remains the reader's responsibility to ensure that these are appropriate for their patients.

Finally, our personal thanks to Jo and Jane.

Peter Barry
Andy Leslie

Foreword

Around the world, intensive care for all age groups has developed at different rates. Within each country, local priorities have governed the way in which services have evolved. In the UK, the equity of health care provision afforded by the National Health Service meant that intensive care technology has spread fairly rapidly and equitably across the whole country. Given the small distances between centres of population, transport was not a major consideration and local enthusiasts have dealt with the issue by employing a variety of solutions. As a result in the country as a whole there are currently hundreds of different transport systems in place.

In other countries local circumstances led to a rather different evolution of the service. For example, in Australia the vast distances between intensive care centres meant that excellent transport facilities were a necessity and as a consequence expert teams with dedicated equipment rapidly emerged. In parts of the USA distance was also an issue. There more flexible funding arrangements made it attractive for health care providers to set up first class services dedicated to transport.

During the last few years a number of new factors have emerged in the UK which have made existing arrangements largely untenable.

Risk

This was highlighted by a road traffic accident which occurred in Northern Region in 1993 involving an ambulance returning to Newcastle with a baby requiring intensive care. In response to this event, the Medical Devices Agency carried out a review of neonatal and paediatric transfers in the UK (the TINA inquiry). The report highlighted various problems. Some of the more important were:

- The standard devices used to secure transport incubators in ambulances were totally inadequate to provide restraint in the event of an accident. Indeed, on closer inspection, it was clear that even if the clamps were able to hold the trolley during an impact, the chassis of the standard ambulance was not.
- It was unreasonable to expect that any transport system weighing more than 200 pounds

(90 kilograms) could be safely carried in a standard ambulance. Some systems in use exceeded 700 pounds (320 kilograms).
- Many additional items of equipment were loaded into the ambulance without any reasonable means of restraint.
- The validity of indemnity arrangements for staff injured in any accident and using such equipment seemed unclear, given that the situation was known to be unsafe.
- Existing Health and Safety legislation regarding manual handling was regularly breached by neonatal transport systems.
- There were no adequate systems for securing the baby in the incubator during the journey.
- Arrangements for staff training were patchy.
- Use of air transport was associated with many additional hazards which appeared to have been fully addressed by only one transport service in the UK.

Although focused on the newborn, most of the problems highlighted by the TINA report were shared by all forms of intensive care transport.

Staffing

The last few years have seen many changes in the working patterns of junior doctors; the high pressure specialities of neonatal and paediatric intensive care have been subject to particularly close regulation. These changes have compounded difficulties regarding the staffing of intensive care retrievals. Only a minority of units have sufficient specialist medical and nursing cover to reliably fill this role and supervise the rest of the service. On the other hand, increased numbers of junior doctors working shorter hours means that providing adequate training is even more complicated.

Demand

During the last five years, neonatal and paediatric intensive care have moved in opposite directions in this regard. For neonatal intensive care, increased numbers of infants cared for in district general hospitals and a falling birth rate have brought a small reduction in the demand for urgent postnatal transfers. This of course compounds the difficulty of those carrying out transports to develop and maintain skill levels.

The same period has seen paediatric intensive care emerge as a speciality in the UK. Therefore at a time of financial stringency both the basic provision for the country and a transport service have had to be established. Since the total number of paediatric intensive care patients is relatively low appropriate catchment populations have been difficult to establish.

Vehicles

As clinical staff, we often take for granted that the local ambulance service will provide a vehicle as and when required. We forget that asking a service with a tight budget to provide a frontline vehicle at random for several hours might pose problems. Similarly, we have on the whole been poor at consulting when we plan to change our transport system for one that might not fit the local vehicles. Where more than one neonatal service exists within the boundaries of a single ambulance trust, they may be requested to transport incubator systems of vastly different configurations. As a result it has been necessary, in some parts of the country, to take the costly step of providing two dedicated vehicles. Conversely, ambulance trusts have, on the whole, not sought the opinion of local intensive care transport teams before ordering new vehicles of a different design. Clearly regular dialogue would go a long way towards helping to resolve these problems.

Conclusions

The overall situation with regard to intensive care transport is quite unsatisfactory, but there are some positive developments on the horizon. Parts of the UK have made a clear decision to provide emergency transfers using a specialist, dedicated service. It is anticipated that transport services of this type will form part of the much heralded new national plan for neonatal intensive care (at the time of writing there has been an official leak of this document but no formal publication). In 2002 the European Union voted to accept new European Standards for transport incubator systems and their carriage in emergency vehicles. Although the UK voted against the new Standards they should become European "Law" in due course. These regulations will place greater responsibilities on those who undertake newborn transfers to ensure that the equipment and procedures used minimise risk for all concerned. However, the specifics around the situation for older children remain largely unregulated.

For those involved in emergency transfer it is important not to ignore the personal responsibility to prepare as thoroughly as possible for the technical and clinical aspects of the task, in order to provide the highest quality of service possible. It is hoped that the material in this book goes some way to achieving that aim.

David Field
Professor of Neonatal Medicine
University of Leicester

Part 1
Planning for safe and effective transport

1 Principles of safe transport

Objectives
This chapter outlines key topics pertinent to establishing and running interhospital transfer services for critically ill infants and children.

Introduction

Services for critically ill infants and children are, to a greater or lesser extent, provided in regionalised patterns, which influence the provision of transport. Many hospitals provide facilities for care of newborn infants of varying levels of intensity where the need for transfer is determined by a requirement for support or treatment beyond that available locally. Babies who are very premature, who require surgery or who are struggling on conventional intensive care are transferred to centres that can provide the necessary support. Locally agreed *in utero* transport policies can avoid the need for intensive care transfer for some of these infants, but a substantial number of postnatal transfers will remain. In the future these may increase as neonatal care is provided in managed clinical networks.

It is now well accepted that the outcome of critical illness or injury in children is better when they are cared for in specialised paediatric intensive care units (PICUs). Such units require high cost equipment and staff and thus cannot be located in all hospitals dealing with children. They are consequently situated in the larger referral centres in countries where PICUs are provided, including the UK. Many hospitals in the UK with emergency paediatric services will thus not have PICU facilities but can, *and will*, from time to time be presented with critically ill children. When critical illness or injury occurs far from a PICU, the child will need admission to and stabilisation in the nearest hospital. If, after stabilisation, the child's needs exceed the facilities of the local hospital, he or she will need to be transported to a referral centre providing intensive care, ideally by the transport team from the PICU. The goal of this team is to function as an extension of the PICU, delivering the same quality of care during transfer.

This chapter gives an outline of all the topics with which this book is concerned. Many of the issues are explored in greater depth elsewhere in the book. The principles of interhospital transfer are outlined here under the following headings:

- Team composition
- Mode of transport
- Setting up a transport programme
- Equipment
- Communication
- Documentation
- Safety
- Transferring a patient.

Team composition

A transport service has organisational and operational teams. Intensive care unit (ICU) staff can be members of either or both. The organisational team (Box 1.1) is made up of senior ICU staff and is tasked with the setting up and management of the transport service. By convention, the service director is a senior ICU consultant and the service coordinator a senior ICU nurse.

Box 1.1 Organisational team tasks

Medical director (PICU, NICU, or A&E consultant)
Oversee programme
Develop policies and protocols
Review/approve equipment and medication lists
Establish and implement outreach programmes
Review transport cases
Manage quality improvement programmes

Transport coordinator (senior nurse)
Develop policies and protocols
Develop/approve equipment and medication lists
Establish and implement outreach programmes
Local liaison (for example, ambulance) and local training
Daily scheduling of transport team members
Review transport cases
Collect transport data (audit)
Manage quality improvement programmes
Budget management

NICU = neonatal intensive care unit; PICU = paediatric intensive care unit.

The operational team is the medic, nurse, paramedic and driver or pilot out on an interhospital patient transfer (Box 1.2). If a child requires only level 1 care it is possible that a nurse, without a medic, may fetch him or her. Critically ill patients require a transport team of at least two personnel, both adequately experienced and accompanied by the ambulance, helicopter or airplane staff. The team leader will usually be a doctor, although advanced neonatal nurse practitioners (ANNPs) are increasingly leading neonatal transports.

Box 1.2   Operational team—qualities and tasks

Transport nurses
Qualities:

- Experienced in PICU or NICU
- Seniority
- Postbasic speciality training plus paediatric and/or neonatal life support
- Availability 24 hours a day, 7 days a week
- Competences:
  management of airways
  operate transport equipment
  understand limits of equipment
  know supplies
  organisaton of transport

Tasks:

- Nursing care of patient during transport
- Liaison with nurses at referring hospital
- Deal sensitively with the family
- Inform the family about patient's destination and how to get there
- Inpatient care after transfer
- Check and restock transport equipment
- Advise transport physician on transport nursing issues

Transport physician (or ANNP)
Qualities:

- Experienced in paediatric/neonatal emergencies and PICU/NICU
- Able to determine diagnostic and therapeutic priorities in critically ill infants and children
- Seniority
- Paediatric and/or neonatal life support
- Available 24 hours a day, 7 days a week
- Competences:
  leadership
  management of airways
  operate transport equipment
  cannulation
  insert IC drains
  can operate within the constraints of the transport environment

Tasks:

- Know bed availability
- Obtain information about patient from the referring team
- Advise about treatment
- Assess need for other specialists, for example, surgeons
- Assess and monitor child's condition

The seniority or grade of the medic and nurse is not an absolute—experience and competence are also considered, as is the patient's diagnosis and perceived condition. In instances of extremely severe illness, it might be prudent if possible to take two senior medics.

The ambulance or aircraft personnel are an integral part of the operational team, and not just drivers. Experienced vehicle personnel, familiar with the needs of the transport team, can save valuable time.

Personnel are the most valuable component of a transport team both in the organisation and the performance of the service.

Mode of transport

Patient transfers are made both within and between hospitals. The principles for the safe and effective movement of a sick patient, particularly where the patient is dependent on support devices such as intravenous pumps and ventilators, apply to any transfer out of the intensive care environment irrespective of the distance needed to travel. Hence, even when a patient is being moved for an investigation or to the operating theatre, the team should adhere to their practised safety procedures.

Three options are available for interhospital patient transfers. The patient may be:

- Sent via the local emergency services
- Sent via the local (referring) emergency medical services, i.e. via ambulance with the referring physician and/or nurse
- Fetched by a specialised critical care transport team.

The first two modes are referred to as one-way transports and the third as two-way transport. The only advantage of sending a patient, or one-way transport, is time. This form of transport has many disadvantages (or two-way transport has many advantages) (Box 1.3).

Interhospital patient transfers are either by road or by air in a helicopter or fixed wing aircraft. Individual intensive care transport teams will have protocols as to which form is used based on various deciding factors. These factors or criteria include:

- Distance between referring and receiving hospital. If the distance exceeds two hours' travel by road, serious consideration has to be given to transferring the patient by helicopter

- Traffic density. This can be partially overcome with the help of the emergency services, including the police who can clear the road. It should not be a reason to summon a helicopter for a short distance
- Buildings in the town or city where the hospitals are located. Transferring a patient to or from a big city by air has the added difficulty of high rise buildings affecting transit and landing
- Weather. Safety is the prime concern in any interhospital patient transfer. There is nothing to be gained from endangering the lives of a helicopter crew and the transport team by sending them out into poor unsafe weather conditions. A timely decision to use an ambulance may save precious time whilst you wait for the weather to clear.

Box 1.3 Advantages of two-way interhospital patient transfers

Entire team—paramedics, nurses, and physicians—have transport training and experience. Outcomes are better for patients transferred by trained teams

Equipment, including critical care equipment like ventilators and monitors, is dedicated for *transporting* critically ill patients

Equipment and drugs are prepared beforehand

Transport team usually from centre where there is staff back up whilst they are away. May even be dedicated transport staff without other responsibilities on that shift

---

Two-way transport (or retrieval) of critically ill patients by trained and experienced staff is the best and most desirable form of interhospital transport.

Setting up a transport programme

A three-pronged approach forms the foundation of success when embarking on an investment of this magnitude—investment not only in financial terms but also in time and commitment. This triad is described below.

Outreach

Identify hospitals in your catchment area and advertise to their relevant staff the proposed or operational service. "Relevant staff" includes the

doctors and nurses in their paediatric department, surgical department, neonatal unit and adult intensive care. A visit to the hospital to talk about the service and deliver laminated posters of the service with a direct dial telephone number to be prominently displayed is arguably the most effective form of this outreach.

Education

Education is necessary at many levels:

- Education programme for the ICU staff who will be doing transfers on transport medicine and interhospital patient transfers
- Study days for staff in referring hospitals on resuscitation and stabilisation of the critically ill child and the needs when preparing for transfer
- Study days for the ambulance staff on the requirements of the service and about emergency paediatrics
- Information to the referring centres on communication lines.

Hard sell

Selling the need for an expensive service is probably the hardest limb of the triad. Professional colleagues outside the ICU and hospital managers and budget holders in your institute need to be convinced of the necessity of such a service. The ICU organisational team need to embark on an exercise of winning the hearts and minds of the colleagues mentioned to ensure that the unit is appropriately staffed and funded. They must know, as must the ICU staff, that "retrieval is not an option but a necessity", that "the ICU can't be seen to pick and choose when they want to help their catchment hospitals", and that the patients in the catchment hospitals are potentially our ICU patients.

Equipment

The operational team must carry all equipment, supplies and drugs necessary for stabilisation and transfer. The team should not rely on the referring hospital for supplies. Paediatric patients are often "held" in adult facilities waiting for the transport team to arrive. These may carry limited paediatric supplies.

The equipment must be regularly checked and serviced. Supplies and drugs (i.e. contents of medical bags) must be replenished after each use; a contents checklist is essential. Checked and restocked boxes and bags should then be sealed, rendering them ready for immediate use. These should be stored in an accessible but protected and restrained space.

There is more in-depth discussion of equipment in chapter 4. The American Critical Care Society lists the equipment needed in transport. Reference to this list can form the template or basis of a transport service's checklist. Essential features of the exhaustive list with guideline recommendations as comments are shown in Box 1.4.

Box 1.4 Equipment required during transport of a critically ill child

Patient movement

- Trolley
- Incubator for children < 5 kg
- Metal pole or shelf system to secure ventilator, pumps, monitors
- Adjustable belts (safety belts) to secure patient in transfer
- Equipment bags: multiple compartments to allow access to individual items without unpacking
- Drug boxes

Airway management

- Equipment to establish and maintain a secure airway
    bag-valve device (for example, Ambu bag) with selected mask sizes
    endotracheal tubes (all sizes), stylet and Magill forceps
    laryngoscope with assorted size blades
- Portable mechanical ventilator
    small, lightweight with economical gas usage
    capable of ventilating infants and children of all ages
    disconnection and high pressure alarms essential
    providing PEEP, facilities for variable Fio_2, I : E ratio, RR, and TV
- Portable oxygen supply
    provide high pressure supply with low pressure metred flow
    sufficient to last duration of transfer with reserve, usually 1–2 hours
- Suction—portable, battery powered

Intravenous infusions

- Equipment to establish and maintain venous and arterial access
- Drugs
    resuscitation drugs

---

    infusions of sedating and paralysing agents (for ventilated patients)
    inotropic infusions
- Infusion pumps—small, lightweight, long battery life

Monitoring

- Monitor:
    portable, battery powered, clear illuminated display
    ECG, oximetry, non-invasive blood pressure, temperature, capnography
    invasive channels (preferably 2) for CVP and invasive BP
    alarms must be *visible* as well as audible because of extraneous noises

Document folder

- Recording chart, audit form, consent form
- Infusion charts and crash drug charts—filled in prior to transfer
- Information for parents, i.e. maps and telephone numbers

Mobile phone
Warm protective clothing for staff

PEEP = positive end expiratory pressure, RR = respiratory rate, TV = tidal volume.

Each transport team, when developing protocols, must devise a list of equipment, supplies and drugs as well as an inventory or checklist.

Communication

When does the ICU take responsibility for the treatment of the critically ill child? The answer to this question is not clear, but once the referring hospital has made contact their referring team is clearly asking for help; however, the arrival of that help will obviously be delayed whilst the operational team is in transit. Interim joint care will be facilitated by communication, so the organisational team must pay particular attention to ensuring ease of communication. Figure 1.1 illustrates some of these issues. Notice that the receiving unit, who will usually be the unit doing the transfer as a two-way transport, have some responsibility for the patient even before they leave base, including responsibilities for assembling a team in a timely fashion and for sending competent staff and appropriate equipment. Notice also that the referring team are substantially responsible for the patient until they hand over to the transport team, and that they continue to have

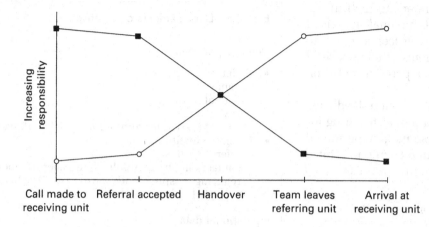

Figure 1.1 Changing levels of responsibility for patient care following referral for transport. (From Brimhall D. The hospital administrators' role. In: MacDonald M, Miller M, eds. *Emergency Transport of the Perinatal Patient.* Toronto: Little, Brown, 1989.)

responsibilities for the patient after transfer: responsibility for assisting the transport team and for notifying the receiving unit of significant laboratory results, such as positive cultures, in the coming hours and days.

Communication has many facets.

- Hotline. A direct line (not through the hospital switchboard) or "hotline" into the ICU that is dedicated to incoming calls (and hence not continuously engaged in a busy ICU) but also open to outgoing national calls will make conversations between consultants considerably easier and more effective. Advertise the number widely in the catchment area.
- Essential information. The ICU must inform their regular referring institutes about the information they will need to ensure that the referring doctor has this essential information to hand when making the telephone call (see below).
- Continuous contact:
  - After a referral has been made there will inevitably be a delay before departure from the receiving hospital. The transport physician or consultant on call should maintain continuous contact by regularly (every half hour) telephoning the referring physician for an update and further advice, if needed. The referring physician should of his or her own volition also maintain continuous contact with updates on any progress, for example child's condition changed making the transfer unnecessary.
  - Once the team has been despatched they must maintain contact with their home

base with a mobile phone throughout the trip, including a brief report about the patient's condition prior to departure for the return journey, expected treatment requirements (for example, ventilator, infusions), and expected time of arrival.

- Inform ambulance crew. The operational team must inform the ambulance crew about the patient's condition and the projected time required for stabilisation and hence expected time of departure for home. This form of communication is particularly important with helicopter crews in air retrievals.
- Talk to staff and family:
  - The referring hospital has asked for help. It is not helpful to arrive with an arrogant "ivory tower" attitude as in most instances the local team will have done a sterling job in difficult circumstances. The referring team will appreciate confirmation and praise as well as measured advice and criticism.
  - The family need relevant information and reassurance, without misplaced optimism. Their child is being taken from them in an ambulance to a strange city, which they might never have visited before. A statement to the effect that the child is very sick but stable and that the team undertakes many transfers successfully every year will provide great comfort. Families have reported that they felt that once the child left it was sure to die. They need to know that that risk is present but small.
- Regular follow up to the referring team and possibly the child's GP as well. Aim to agree to

return the patient to the referring institute as soon as he or she has had maximal benefit of the ICU. This allows convalescence close to the patient's family, promotes efficient use of ICU beds, and advances cooperation between institutes.

- Feedback. The ICU must provide feedback, particularly about stabilisation, as teaching for the referring institute personnel. A period of secondment by nurses from referring institutes to the ICU could also serve this purpose.

> Communication, communication, communication

Documentation

A good doctor or nurse is only as good as the records he or she keeps. A clear and concise written clinical record is important with any patient treatment, but possibly more important during interhospital patient transfers as these are patients who are usually critically ill and who in addition, for the duration of the transfer, are not managed in an optimal environment. Important features of this transport documentation are:

- It provides the only patient record for the duration of the transfer
- Essential link between the referring facility, transport team, and the receiving facility
- Documentary evidence of the course of patient evaluation, treatment, and changes in condition
- Basis for planning the patient's care and case review
- Permanent health record.

Box 1.5 lists the essential elements for inclusion in a transport log. Further examples of transport documentation are given in Appendix 1.

> A good doctor or nurse is only as good as the records he or she keeps.

Safety

The safe return of the operational team is a presumption that is made without daring to contemplate any other alternative. However, interhospital patient transfers are a high risk activity, so safety considerations are important at all times. Safety is not only about the avoidance of accidents; it also considers the physical

---

Box 1.5 Data elements of a transport log

Demographic data

- Patient:
  name
  date of birth
  sex
  weight (*very important for drug calculations*)
- Referring institute:
  referring physician
  contact telephone number and pager number
  referring hospital and ward or unit where patient will be located

Operational data

- Staff member receiving call
- Times:
  of receiving call
  of embarkation
  of arrival at referring hospital
  of departure from referring hospital
  of arrival at ICU at receiving hospital

Clinical data

- Predeparture:
  brief incident-related history, provisional diagnosis, reason for transfer request
  initial vital signs and pertinent physical findings
  relevant laboratory results, for example, arterial blood gas (ABG)
  treatment given, for example, ventilator settings, infusions, antibiotics
  recommendations given
- Assessment on arrival at referring hospital:
  clinical findings by transport team, including treatment, for example, ventilator settings
  recent laboratory investigations, for example, ABG, CXR with ETT position
  interventions at referring hospital
- In transit:
  vital signs (monitoring) during transfer
  medication administered by transport team
  problems encountered and treatment given
- On return to PICU:
  vital signs
  ventilator settings

Checklists

- For referring hospital
- Predeparture (*focuses on equipment needed*)
- Prereturn (*focuses on patient care*)

---

wellbeing of the team and legal and clinical governance aspects in transfers (Box 1.6).

Two points about safety merit further comment.

1. *Ambulance speed.* If the referring hospital has the ability to stabilise a sick patient, which all should do, and if your patient is stabilised

before returning, in most instances there is no additional benefit to the patient in saving a few minutes' travel time by travelling under blue light conditions. This is balanced by the many disadvantages of high speed travel, such as increased movement of the back of the ambulance possibly placing an airway at risk and definitely making any intervention more difficult, increased anxiety of the operational team in an already difficult situation, and increased risk of an accident. Travelling at high speed and weaving through traffic is almost never necessary and should be discouraged.

2. *Passenger safety.* The physical safety of the operational team is as important as the patient. There is no sense in endangering the team by travelling fast for the perceived benefit of the patient.

> Speed kills—even in an ambulance

Box 1.6 Safety considerations during transfers

Organisational

- Clinical protocols
- Operational protocols and checklists
- Regular team training
- Audit
- Insurance

Passenger safety

- Patient and all transport team members must wear safety belts or other restraints
- All equipment must be secured to trolley, for example, ventilator, oxygen cylinders, pumps
- Loose objects, such as drug and equipment bags, should be strapped in when in the ambulance
- The ambulance should obey the speed limit and traffic signals unless there are compelling clinical reasons to do otherwise

Patient safety

- Predeparture checklist
- Crash chart
- Careful monitoring throughout transfer

Transport team safety

- Warm clothing
- Travel sickness tablets
- Nutrition
  the transport team should not miss meals
  high calorie snacks should be available in transit
- Money and credit cards carried for emergencies

Transporting a patient

This section deals with a retrieval step by step and will thus of necessity repeat principles outlined previously. It is not meant to be a didactic description of a transfer but rather highlights aspects regarded as important.

Referral

Interhospital patient transfers require excellent communication between the referring hospital, the operational team, and their receiving ICU. This communication begins with the initial telephone call and ends when the patient is admitted to the receiving ICU. The initial call may be an actual referral or a request for advice, the latter a facility or service the ICU must advertise to its clientele.

In the event of a referral the ICU may or may not be able to accept the patient. Should the ICU be unable to accept the transfer the consultant should advise his/her referring colleague what the situation is and the outlook for a potential bed in the near future. Alternative arrangements could be referral to another ICU or holding the child in the referring institute's neonatal or adult ICU until a bed is available in the accepting ICU. In paediatrics the national bed bureau has a record of ICU bed availability nationwide that is kept up to date, and there are some similar local schemes in neonatal care. Communication about respective bed occupancy between neighbouring ICUs is thus necessary to be able to give referring hospitals useful information as to who to contact.

When a patient is accepted, from the outset the ICU team must assess the equipment and medication needs of the individual patient. This can only be achieved by obtaining relevant information, which must include:

- Brief incident-related history
- Current vital signs
- Child's weight
- Pertinent physical findings
- Relevant laboratory results and
- Treatment modalities instituted.

The unit transport log is used to record details and will act as the patient's clinical record until admission to the ICU. This standard form will guide the doctor or nurse taking the call to obtain *all* the important information and later direct the team as they prepare. As the responsibility of the receiving hospital begins when the referring institute makes the initial contact, it is very important to have accurate documentation of *all* communication, i.e. recommendations of care must be recorded.

Team composition

The on-call consultant has to make decisions regarding staffing the transport based on the reported condition of the patient and the experience of his or her resident staff. It can often be difficult to determine the condition of a patient over the telephone. The referring doctor might be inexperienced and through anxiety exaggerate the patient's severity or through inexperience underassess how sick the child really is. The safest advice is to anticipate a more rather than a less severe scenario.

While a small number of acute transfers may be undertaken by a nurse alone, most will require two people. As discussed above, the team leader will usually be a doctor, though in neonates an ANNP may assume this role. Whoever leads the transfer must be able to deal with the worst scenario that can be reasonably projected, including sudden deterioration of the patient during the journey. Consideration must be given to whether the doctor or ANNP is experienced enough to undertake the retrieval without the support of a consultant and to whether the situation warrants more than one doctor or nurse.

Stabilisation

Stabilisation by the referring team is focused on maintenance of airway, breathing, and circulation. Before transport all patients must have a stable airway, adequate ventilation, and vascular access. If any of these is recognised to be deficient at the initial call, the referring hospital has to have the capability of intervention: the basics of airway maintenance, ventilation, and vascular access should be available at all facilities that provide care to children. Other interventions such as drug therapy (for example, antibiotics, anticonvulsants, sedation) and tube placement (for example, urinary catheter, NG tubes) could be advised.

A stable patient will not only improve outcome but also quicken turnaround time.

> Stabilisation begins at the referring hospital. A retrieval service is not a resuscitation service.

Stabilise or scoop and run?

It is a general principle of transportation of critically ill patients that they should be stabilised prior to transfer. Adequate control of the airway, breathing, and circulation should be established, and treatment should be optimised to ensure that the patient is in the best possible condition for transfer. Sometimes, however, the patient has a *time critical condition* where delaying specialist treatment such as neurosurgery or extracorporeal life support (ECMO) is actually dangerous. In these situations a judgement must be made concerning the risk of transport against the risk of denying the patient specialist treatment. The key to this decision is the assessment of the patient's current treatment, and whether any treatment that you can give can stabilise the patient. A good example of a patient who should be transferred quickly is a patient with an expanding intracranial haematoma that is beyond the skill of local surgeons, who is already paralysed, ventilated with low-normal $Pa\text{co}_2$ and has received mannitol. Such a patient needs urgent neurosurgery, not further intensive care. The opposite situation could be a patient with sepsis who has not received adequate fluid resuscitation, where a few hours spent stabilising the patient is likely to lead to improvement and make transport much safer.

> *Always stabilise the patient before transfer; unless:*
> There is nothing you can do to improve the patient's condition
> The benefits of treatment at the base hospital outweigh the risks of transfer
> The parents are fully aware of the risks and benefits and accept them.

Operational team assessment and management

In the transport setting, urgent treatment and the management of life-threatening problems are the priority. Evaluations that are diagnosis specific may not be necessary until returning to the ICU. Although the whole patient must be assessed, examination in depth should be deferred until after the transport; for example, a 2-year-old child who has ingested tablets need not have an ear examination in transit.

When the transport team arrive, their priorities are:

- A rapid assessment of the patient, focusing on A, B, and C

- To receive current information from the referring team
- To review *x* ray films and laboratory tests
- To secure all lines and tubes before loading the patient.

Airway and breathing

The airway must be patent and stable for the duration of the entire transfer. If in any doubt about the need to ventilate or intubate the patient to secure his or her airway, it is preferable to intubate before departure. If the patient is already intubated and ventilating adequately, elective reintubation to, for example, change from an orotracheal to a nasotracheal tube is not necessary. In a well sedated and/or paralysed patient an oral tube can be safely secured and maintained.

- Infants:

  - Continuous monitoring with oximetry and transcutaneous gases are advised.
  - Ventilation should, in most instances, aim to maintain Pao_2 at 6–10 kPa and $Paco_2$ at 4·0–6·0 kPa. Use higher oxygen concentrations and higher ventilator rates than the patient would require when not in transit, but avoid hyperoxia and hypocarbia.
  - Sedate babies for transfer and use muscle relaxation if sedation is not sufficient to settle the patient.

- Older children:

  - Continuous monitoring with oximetry and capnometry are advised.
  - Ventilation should aim to maintain Pao_2 at more than 13 kPa and $Paco_2$ at less than 4·0–4·5 kPa. Use higher oxygen concentrations and higher ventilator rates than the patient would require when not in transit.
  - Patients who are intubated should be sedated and *paralysed* for the duration of the transfer.

Circulation

- Patients must have one secure vascular access *at least*. This would suffice for a high dependency patient who is self-ventilating. In ventilated patients on continuous infusions of sedatives and paralysing agents more than one venous line is necessary.

- Fluid resuscitation can be done en route but must have been initiated before departure.
- If inotropes are necessary, start infusion before moving.

Neurological status

Evaluation of the level of consciousness is an ongoing assessment performed at the same time as A, B, and C. Consider airway protection if the level of consciousness is low.

- Infants:

  - Assess and record all seizures.
  - Consider specific treatment for encephalopathic babies.

- Older children:

  - If the child is responsive, ask the parents whether the behaviour is appropriate.
  - Assess and record all seizures.
  - ALWAYS check the pupils on arrival and before departure. Ensure that you corroborate your findings with the referring staff if there are concerns, for example unreactive pupils, and that you communicate these concerns with the parents before you move the patient.
  - Consider specific treatment if raised intracranial pressure is suspected.

Temperature control

The smaller the patient, the more likely it is that temperature control will be a major element of the transfer process. A small infant has a high ratio of surface area to body mass, which encourages rapid heat loss. Heat loss increases oxygen consumption by increasing the metabolic rate. This can lead to lactic acidosis and even hypoxia. Poor post-transfer temperature is a better predictor of death in premature infants than gestation or birthweight.

Monitor the temperature continuously—preferably core temperature in infants, toddlers, and unconscious patients. A high temperature also increases metabolic demands. Loss of temperature can occur:

- With the initial event, i.e. severe illness, knocked down in street
- With exposure for evaluation and management
- During procedures

- With movement from one environment to another.

Standard warming devices should be available at the referring hospital:

- Infants:
  - Incubator for infants weighing less than 5 kilograms
  - Covering the head
  - Warming mattress.
- Older children:
  - Space blanket.

Head-to-toe examination

A brief head-to-toe examination, particularly in the unconscious patient, may alert the transport team to problems not already identified. Document any unusual bruises, rashes, or skin markings. Look for congenital abnormalities in the newborn.

Miscellaneous interventions

- Place a gastric tube (oral or nasal) if the patient is intubated or if there is abdominal distension and leave on free drainage.
- A urinary catheter is appropriate in shocked patients to document urine output.
- Assay the blood sugar—especially in young children.
- Keep the patient nil by mouth—may have motion sickness.

Talking to the parents

Parents should wait at the referring hospital until the transport team arrives. This will allow the transport team to:

- Obtain further history:
  - Obstetric and perinatal
  - Immunisations
  - Allergies
  - Past medical history, including medications
  - Recent exposure to communicable diseases
- Inform or update the parents about the child's condition
- Obtain any consents.

Should a parent accompany the child (and the operational team) in the ambulance? There is no advice or guidance on this issue, so practices of transport teams are based on personal biases and experience as well as practical considerations.

- Is there space? Is there a spare seat?
- Does the mother have ongoing obstetric needs that the transport team are not qualified to attend to?
- Will the presence of a parent impair patient care?
- Is the parent at risk of travel sickness, given that he or she is anxious about his or her child and is travelling in an unfamiliar way, i.e. facing sideways in the back of an ambulance? How will the operational team cope with a sick vomiting parent and the sick child?
- Is the ambulance insured to carry a passenger not a patient?

Predeparture check

Before leaving the transport physician and nurse should go through a predeparture checklist. This list must require them to tick off item by item and is part of the transport log. An example is given in the documentation appendix (see Appendix 1).

Monitoring

It is almost impossible to examine a patient in the back of an ambulance or a helicopter. It is consequently essential that the patient is monitored, that the monitor is resistant to movement interference, and that it has a screen visible in all light conditions. The parameters monitored will depend on the degree of invasive treatment (for example, intubated or not) and monitoring (for example, intra-arterial cannula present). Aside from heart rate with a visible ECG, oxygen saturation, temperature, and blood pressure as standard minimums for all patients, the operational team may also monitor invasive blood pressure or central venous pressure and end-tidal CO_2 where these are available.

End-tidal CO_2 is a parameter that is not widely monitored in children in the ICU, possibly because of the relatively high cost of the equipment. It is, however, an extremely useful and probably essential parameter in interhospital patient transfers. It gives the operational team a breath by breath record of the patient's ventilatory status and hence the integrity of the ventilator, tubing, endotracheal tube, and lungs. It is so easy to disconnect a tube with patient movement onto the trolley or into the incubator, or with movement of the ambulance. This disconnection may not be noticed by inspection for chest movement, as this is extremely difficult in a

Box 1.7 Postreturn assessment

On arrival back in ICU

Observations: HR:_____   BP: ___ / ___ mmHg   Cap. refill _____ secs

Temperature: Core:_____°C   Peripheral:_____°C

Ventilation: Rate:_____ PIP:_____ PEEP:_____

$\qquad\qquad$ Fio$_2$:_____ Ti:_____ Te:_____ I : E:_____

ABG on portable vent: pH:_____ P_{CO_2}:_____ P_{O_2}:_____

$\qquad\qquad\qquad$ HCO$_3$:_____ BE:_____ Sao_2:_____

$\qquad\qquad\qquad$ Glucose:_____

Pupils: Left:_____   Right:_____

Urine output during transfer:_____ ml/kg/h

Ti = inspiratory time, Te = expiratory time, I : E = inspiratory : expiratory ratio.

moving ambulance, but will instantaneously be recognised by an alarming end-tidal CO_2 monitor.

A written record of the patient's vital signs must be recorded in a flow sheet in the transport log. This record should start prior to moving the patient, continue throughout the journey, and discontinue when the patient is attached to the monitor in the receiving ICU. The flow sheet should also have the facility to record all treatment en route. This is the only documentary evidence between hospitals of the patient's condition, treatment, changes in condition, and adverse events. It can form the basis for planning the current patient's care, case review, and audit. Examples are given in Appendix 1.

Postreturn assessment

On arrival in the receiving ICU, the operational team must make a brief assessment prior to admitting the patient to an ICU bed. This is essentially to draw a line between the transfer and the arrival, in the same manner as the team ensured that they monitored the patient before departing and communicated any concerns with the referring team. This assessment is recorded on the transport log (Box 1.7).

Summary
Safe transport can be encapsulated in the following key points:

- Communication
- Planning
- Correct team composition
- Continuous stabilisation
- Careful and continuous assessment
- Monitoring and recording throughout
- Consideration for staff and parents
- Complete, accurate and legible documentation
- SAFETY.

2 Transport physiology

Apart from the hazards of equipment failure and medical staff having to work in a strange environment, interhospital transfer imposes a number of other physiological stresses on the patient. These can have an unpredictable effect on the cardiovascular system, causing hypo- or hypertension, and may also adversely affect other systems, such as acutely raising intracerebral pressure during deceleration. These physical stresses may be dynamic, as in acceleration or deceleration, or static, relating to the problems of the ambulance environment (see chapter 3) or factors such as noise, vibration, and temperature.

Objectives
To understand some of the physiological effects associated with interhospital transport.
To know the strategies that may be employed to minimise these effects.
To understand basic altitude physiology.

Acceleration and deceleration

Rapid acceleration and deceleration can lead to pooling of blood, with sudden variations in venous return to the heart and subsequent changes in cardiac output. The Starling curve, which plots stroke volume against end diastolic volume, gives an idea of some of the effects that may be encountered (Fig. 2.1). The normal curve (curve 1) shows an increase in cardiac output with increasing filling pressure, up to a point where the myocardium fails, and no further increase, or a reduction is seen. In the failing heart, or the normal heart in hypervolaemia, increases in filling pressure are not accompanied by an increase in cardiac output (curve 2).

If the patient is lying, as is typical, with the head towards the front of the ambulance, rapid acceleration will tend to reduce venous return, and hence reduce filling pressure, leading to reduced cardiac output. Conversely, deceleration increases venous return to the heart and may increase cardiac output, or in the failing heart, may cause heart failure and reduced cardiac output. In general, the patient will tolerate sudden increases in venous return better than sudden decreases. Hypovolaemia should be corrected before transfer, if possible. After clinical examination, volume status is best assessed by observing the response to small (3–5 ml/kg), rapidly infused (2–3 minutes) boluses of crystalloid, such as normal saline 0·9%. In the normovolaemic patient, a short-lived rise in filling pressure is seen, accompanied by an improvement in cardiac output (Fig. 2.2, curve 2). If hypovolaemia is present, there is little change in filling pressure or cardiac output (Fig. 2.2, curve 1). Hypervolaemia is relatively uncommon in the clinical situations covered in this manual. A sustained rise in filling pressure in response to a fluid challenge, with no change or a deterioration in cardiac output (Fig. 2.2, curve 3),

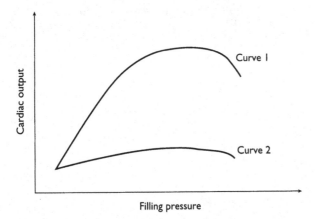

Figure 2.1 The relationship between stroke volume and end diastolic volume for the normal heart (curve 1) and the failing heart (curve 2). (Adapted from Lawler PG. Transfer of critically ill patients: Part 2—preparation for transfer. *Care Crit Ill* 2000;16:94–7 with permission.)

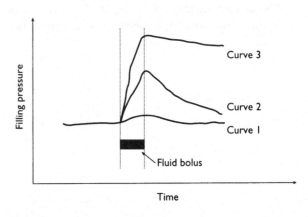

Figure 2.2 The change in filling pressure in response to fluid challenge. (Adapted from Lawler PG. Transfer of critically ill patients: Part 2—preparation for transfer. *Care Crit Ill* 2000;16:94–7 with permission.)

suggests hypervolaemia or myocardial depression. Treatment may include inotropic and ventilatory support and diuresis. It should be emphasised that hypervolaemia is much less common, and better tolerated, than hypovolaemia in most clinical situations.

One case in which the emphasis is slightly different is the newborn or preterm infant. Because of the relative stiffness of the ventricular wall, fluid loading is not well tolerated, and increasing heart rate is relatively more important as a mechanism for increasing cardiac output.

Normally patients respond to sustained changes in filling pressure by altering heart rate. A sudden decrease in venous pressure leads to tachycardia and a sudden increase to bradycardia. Critically ill patients may have poor baroreceptor function and dysautonomia, which reduce their ability to compensate in this way.

In practice, acceleration is rarely a problem in an ambulance or aircraft. Even at take off, forces of less than 0·25 G are experienced during commercial flights, and only around 0·5 G on landing. However, rapid braking in an ambulance can produce forces equivalent to 7 G, which can have serious, albeit transient, effects on the patient. This is another reason for ensuring that the return journey with the patient is made at normal road speed with minimum changes in speed.

Pulmonary blood flow is also affected by motion changes. In acceleration (assuming the patient to be lying head first), blood is diverted towards the lung base, and away from the anatomical apex. In deceleration the reverse is true. This may worsen ventilation–perfusion mismatch.

Similar effects happen with sudden side to side movements, and if the patient has unilateral lung disease; for instance, changes in oxygenation that occur when turning corners may contribute to patient instability.

Changes caused by movement of large organs and the diaphragm

The abdomen and thorax are separated by the diaphragm, and acceleration or deceleration will displace the abdominal contents and hence move the diaphragm. Again, depending upon the orientation of the patient, this will either increase or reduce lung volume, and may lead to underventilation, hypercapnia, and hypoxia.

Changes in intracranial pressure

Sudden increases in venous pooling in the head will lead to increases in intracranial pressure, which may be of significance to the head injured patient. Also, acute reductions in blood pressure caused by venous pooling in the legs will reduce cerebral perfusion (Fig. 2.3).

Specific considerations apply to transferring patients in helicopters. Ideally the patient should be positioned across the direction of travel, or their position should be changed depending on whether acceleration or deceleration is likely (Fig. 2.4). In practice, neither of these options is possible, and the best way to avoid problems with acceleration and deceleration is to travel in a controlled manner.

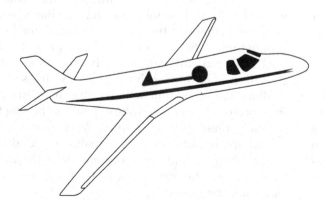

Figure 2.3 Fixed wing aircraft fly "nose up". Patients positioned in the head first position (shown here) are at risk—feet first or transverse is safer. (From Lawler PG. Transfer of critically ill patients: Part 2—preparation for transfer. *Care Crit Ill* 2000;16:94–7 with permission.)

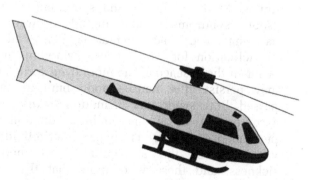

Figure 2.4 Rotary wing aircraft fly "head down/tail up". The patient is best positioned with the head in the direction of travel (as shown). (From Lawler PG. Transfer of critically ill patients: Part 2—preparation for transfer. *Care Crit Ill* 2000;16:94–7 with permission.)

Noise and vibration

High noise levels are commonplace in both aeromedical and road transfers, with noise levels of 95 dB being recorded inside some helicopters. This can be disconcerting to the patient, increasing anxiety and cardiovascular instability. Noise levels as low as 70 dB have been associated with changes in heart rate and peripheral vasoconstriction in preterm infants. Incubators also have high levels of ambient noise. Ear protection should be routinely used for patients, and is necessary for staff during noisy retrievals, such as in a helicopter.

Noise will also make audible alarms ineffective and therefore these should have a visual component as well. Auscultation with a stethoscope is impossible in a noisy environment.

Vibration may also upset the patient, worsening feelings of nausea and motion sickness. High levels of vibration may increase the risk of intracranial bleeding in preterm infants, although the evidence for this is not good. Greatest vibration is experienced during take off and landing of aircraft. The use of gel filled mattresses has been shown to reduce vibration during transport in a neonatal model. Whether this has any effect in improving patient outcome is unknown.

Vibration will also disturb some monitors such as non-invasive blood pressure monitors and pulse oximeters.

Motion sickness will occur in up to 50% of the transport team, and an unknown number of transported patients. The most overt form of motion sickness is characterised by nausea, sweating, and vomiting. The symptoms may be severe enough to incapacitate the team member and prevent him or her from undertaking their duties. More subtle are the symptoms of the "sopite syndrome", which include drowsiness, yawning, decreased mental agility, and a disinclination for work. These symptoms may occur in the absence of the more overt form, and may persist after nausea and vomiting have passed. Both syndromes of motion sickness are accompanied by a measurable reduction in performance. There is huge interindividual variability in the susceptibility to motion sickness, and those who know that they are susceptible should consider the use of antiemetic preparations, with the caveat that these may also induce drowsiness. Biofeedback methods and relaxation techniques have also been shown to be effective in the treatment or prevention of motion sickness.

Temperature changes

Problems with thermal regulation are discussed in chapter 6 and are of most relevance to the neonatal patient. However, older children and infants may also suffer from thermal stress, and frequent monitoring of temperature is necessary.

Heat is lost from the body by four mechanisms.

1. Convection. Air currents replace warm air near the body with cold air, which is warmed by convection from the skin, and the body cools as it loses energy. The chilling power of the wind can produce extreme cooling.
2. Conduction is the transfer of heat between solids in contact. As the area of contact between the patient and the cold environment is normally small, this is a less important cause of heat loss.
3. Radiation. The transfer of heat by electromagnetic energy, such as sunshine, or from the patient to a cold surface.
4. Evaporation. Water evaporation uses energy, resulting in heat loss from the skin when sweat evaporates, and from the respiratory tract, where air is warmed and humidified. The low humidity of ambient air during long fixed wing retrievals may increase heat and water loss.

If a patient needs to produce more heat, they will need to use more oxygen. The amount of oxygen will depend on the amount of heat loss. It can be seen that children who are not adequately warmed will need to increase their cardiac output in order to deliver the oxygen required for heat production. This is often not a problem in well children but can severely exacerbate the condition of children who are already shocked.

Many larger infants will be able to maintain their body temperature at the expense of having to increase their cardiac output. Very small and premature infants are often unable to produce sufficient heat and may become hypothermic. This causes the double insult of exacerbated shock and hypothermia.

A "thermoneutral" environment is one in which additional cardiac output is not required to maintain temperature. It is important to understand that this will be a higher temperature

Table 2.1 The effect of increasing altitude on alveolar PA_{O_2}. (Reproduced with permission from Jainovich DG. *Handbook of Paediatric and Neonatal Transport Medicine.* Hanley and Belfus, 1996)

Pa_{CO_2} (kPa)	PA_{O_2} (kPa) (assuming $Fi_{O_2} = 0.21$)		PA_{O_2} (kPa) (assuming $Fi_{O_2} = 1.0$)	
	At 760 mmHg	At 500 mmHg	At 760 mmHg	At 500 mmHg
2.5	16.5	10	91.2	66
5.3	13.2	6.5	88	64
8	10	3.3	66	61

Table 2.2 Barometric pressure and approximate gas volumes at different altitudes (Reproduced with permission from Jainovich DG. *Handbook of Paediatric and Neonatal Transport Medicine.* Hanley and Belfus, 1996)

Altitude (m)	Barometric pressure (mmHg)	Atmospheres	Relative volume
Sea level	760	1.0	1.0
1500 (unpressurised aircraft may fly at this altitude)	630	0.83	1.2
2500 (commercial flights pressurised to this altitude)	560	0.77	1.3
5000	380	0.5	2.0

than that required to maintain an infant's body temperature.

The retrieval team should minimise heat loss by wrapping the patient up appropriately, while still allowing access to the patient for monitoring, etc. The head is a major source of heat loss and should be covered by a hat or blanket.

Chemical warming packs may be used to warm blankets and sheets, but should not be placed directly against the patient. Warming with surgical gloves filled with hot water poses a serious risk of scalding and should not be used.

Atmospheric pressure

Barometric pressure changes on ascent to altitude are covered in chapter 5. Two problems arise that are of importance to the retrieval team.

Expansion of gas filled spaces

This can cause a small undrained pneumothorax to become a large tension pneumothorax.

Pneumothoraces should be drained prior to undertaking an air retrieval.

Air in other body cavities, such as the stomach, will expand and may interfere with ventilation or predispose to vomiting and aspiration. It should be drained with a nasogastric tube left on free drainage. A syndrome known (in the USA) as "high altitude flatus explosion" may also prove problematic.

Blood pressure cuffs and air filled bandages or splints may be affected and should be loosened. Endotracheal tube cuffs will also expand and should be deflated or filled with an appropriate volume of saline instead of air.

On descent eustachian tube dysfunction may be a cause of severe earache and sinus pain may also occur.

Reduction in oxygen tension

Oxygen tension falls with altitude, and can be calculated from the alveolar gas equation:

$$PA_{O_2} = (BP - P_{H_2O}) \times Fi_{O_2} (P_{CO_2} \times 1/R)$$

where BP is the barometric pressure, and R the respiratory quotient. Table 2.1 shows the effect of increasing altitude on alveolar P_{O_2}.

Even in "pressurised" aircraft the inspired oxygen tension will need to be increased, as the cabin is only pressurised to approximately 2500 m, and an oxygen concentration of 30% is needed to maintain inspired P_{O_2} at the same level as on the ground. Apart from this, the effects of hypobaria are limited by the pressurisation of commercial airliners, and the fact that unpressurised aircraft such as helicopters do not normally fly very high. Problems may occur if the patient is already receiving 100% oxygen at sea level, or if the geography of an area means that substantial ascent needs to be made. Table 2.2 gives the barometric pressure and approximate gas volumes at different altitudes.

Summary
Acceleration and deceleration in the transport environment lead to cardiorespiratory instability and should be minimised where possible.
The adverse effects of motion are worse in patients who are hypovolaemic, and hypovolaemia should be actively sought and treated.
Neonates tolerate fluid boluses less well than older patients. This does not mean that hypovolaemia is better tolerated, just that greater caution is needed when fluid challenging the neonatal patient.
Noise and vibration are common in the transport environment and may provoke cardiovascular instability. Noise protection should be routinely used for patients.
Motion sickness is common and may impair the performance of the transport team. Subtle symptoms include drowsiness and decreased performance.
The physiological problems caused by hypoxia at altitude and expansion of air spaces and body parts should be understood and anticipated.

3 The ambulance environment

Objectives
This chapter is concerned with transfers in ground ambulances, both planning for transport and the practicalities of working in ambulances. It is important to appreciate the safety-focused legislative frameworks that cover ambulance transfers, as well as understanding the constraints imposed on practice by the environment.

Introduction

The period of a transfer when the patient is at highest risk is the time spent in transit and this is also when the attending staff feel the most exposed and vulnerable. This is because ambulances are not intensive care units. If there is a clinical emergency more expert personnel are not at hand to help. If a monitor or ventilator fails there isn't a store room to get another from. Power and gas supplies can run out. All of this, plus the challenges of working in a cramped, moving environment with variable light and heat, means that ambulances impose some serious challenges for transport clinicians.

Nearly all transfers use ambulances. If aeromedical transport is utilised, an ambulance will usually still be required to transport the team and equipment from the aircraft landing site to the receiving hospital. An ambulance may also be utilised as a back up if aeromedical transfer is not possible. Aeromedical teams also need to consider the compatibility of aircraft trolley systems with ground ambulances at both ends of the journey.

The aim, as outlined in the Paediatric Intensive Care Society's "Paediatric Intensive Care Standards", should be to recreate intensive care for the child within the ambulance, to "provide intensive care on the move". Although this chapter discusses issues in the planning and design of transport vehicles, it must be borne in mind that these are all only as good as the personnel using them. The "Transport of Neonates in Ambulances (TINA)" report highlighted this issue, recommending that teams "should ensure that suitably skilled staff, together with equipment and vehicles are available to ensure the demands of neonatal transport are met efficiently".

Standards and reports

There are several documents that have specific implications for the way transport ambulances are configured, and some of the important features of these are outlined here. Not all of these refer to all kinds of ambulance transfer.

Although some European standards are not law at present, they will have that status in the future. Even though equipment is not available to fully comply with some of these, they represent a goal for future practice that should be worked towards. Individual centres must each assess the risk of the equipment they use and the vehicles they use it in.

European Standard for transport incubator systems (CEN 13976-2, draft)

This draft document from the European Union Standards Committee has been accepted and will become binding in due course.

Key issues are likely to be:

- Maximum incubator system weight, probably 140 kg
- Users must purchase complete transport systems, and not modify them
- Incubator systems should be secured in ambulances by two separate devices, each capable of restraining the incubator in the event of a sudden 10 G deceleration. This is, very approximately, equivalent to coming to a dead stop from 30 mph (50 kmph).

Equipment is not available from manufacturers at this time that allows users to completely comply with these regulations and so there is likely to be a derogation period while such equipment is developed. As soon as the document is formally published those responsible for producing and operating transport incubator systems need to be working towards producing a system that will provide a safe environment within the ambulance, particularly in the light of the safety and restraint regulations. Restraint is discussed further, below.

Two other standards are relevant. One is concerned with stretchers used in ambulances (CEN EN 1865) and one covers medical vehicles and their equipment (CEN 1789). Although neither is specifically concerned with neonatal or paediatric transfer, they emphasise security and restraint as key issues. All the standard stretcher trolleys used in ambulances are regulated by these standards. Although some stretchers meet the standard, such as the Falcon (Ferno, Bradford, UK), any modifications undertaken to convert them to paediatric intensive care (PIC) trolleys will not. Thus paediatric transfer trolleys are relatively unregulated, especially when compared to the new incubator regulations, but the key messages about weight limitation and restraint in the vehicle should not go unheeded.

> European legislation will increasingly determine standards for transport equipment.

Ambulance configuration

The design and layout of the ambulance cabin may help improve on some of the limitations of the transport environment. Increasingly, ambulance services are finding that their operational needs are best met by providing dedicated vehicles for transport teams. These are discussed in more detail below. For this reason it is worth being aware of some of the major considerations in designing such a vehicle. Design is substantially limited by space. The typical ambulance has about 7 m^2 of floor space, compared to the recommended standard of 25 m^2 for an intensive care unit (ICU) bed space.

Trolley and seating positions

Trolleys, either with incubators or without, may be mounted transversely or longitudinally, and this substantially determines the seating plan (Figs 3.1, 3.2). Both positions have some advantages. The transverse position is more stable, as the weight of the trolley is not concentrated on one side of the vehicle. The personnel are seated facing the direction of travel, which reduces motion sickness. The transverse position will be the preferred option for neonatal incubators in the European Standard. The longitudinal position allows central mounting of the trolley and so access to both sides of the patient. In both configurations the numbers and precise orientations of seats may vary.

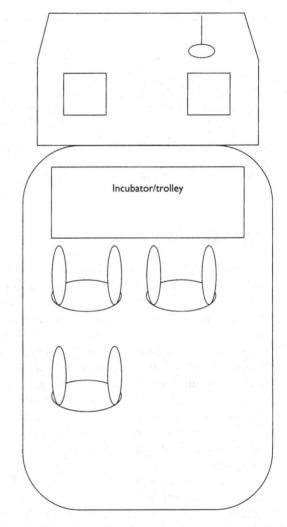

Figure 3.1 Transverse incubator/trolley mounting. Note the passengers are facing the direction of travel.

Seating configurations should allow one person to sit at the head of a child on a trolley to provide constant clinical monitoring and management of the airway, though for neonates a position that allows observation of the baby in the incubator may be preferable. The second member of the team needs to be in a position that will enable him or her to have continuous viewing of the monitor and easy access to additional equipment. Anyone else, such as a parent, who may be present must be properly secured.

Power

Ambulances should be designed with reliable robust electrical systems for the provision of power to lights, heaters, air conditioning and

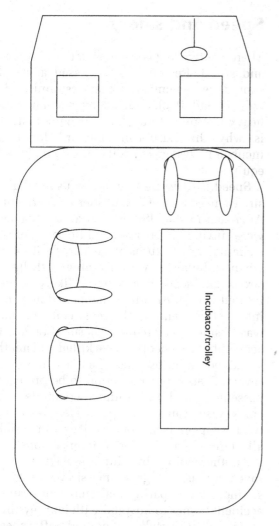

Figure 3.2 Longitudinal incubator/trolley mounting. It may be possible to mount the incubator more centrally.

communications systems. It is desirable for transport teams to utilise ambulance power to conserve the batteries of the transport equipment. As ambulance power supplies are generated by the movement of the vehicle, this is a good option and should be widely used. Ensure when connecting to the ambulance power supply that the ambulance engine is running, in order to avoid ambulance battery failure.

Transport incubators have traditionally been configured to allow them to take power from the vehicle. The problem for other items of equipment, such as pumps and monitors, has been that they have been designed to take external power from only alternating current (AC) sources and ambulance power is usually direct current (DC).

There are two possible solutions to this problem. Firstly, some equipment is now being made that can run on an external DC supply, and secondly the ambulance may be fitted with a power "inverter" which converts the usual DC supply to AC. It is to be hoped that the future standardisation of transport equipment across Europe will resolve these issues so that transport teams do not risk battery failure in essential equipment.

Heating

Temperature within the ambulance environment will be variable and seasonal. There will also be temperature changes during transfer of the patient from the unit to the ambulance. Additional warmth may be achieved by the ambulance temperature control system, incubator temperature control, or a chemically activated warming mattress.

Although the UK climate is mostly miserably nondescript, it is highly desirable for ambulances to have both effective heating for very cold conditions and air conditioning for very warm days. The cabin should be secure against rain and wind. Staff also need to wear appropriate clothing, which will also allow them to work comfortably. Taking several layers allows you to move comfortably from icy conditions while loading the vehicle to very hot conditions in the cabin in transit.

Lighting

It should be possible to incrementally and rapidly adjust cabin lighting from low levels that may be appropriate at night on the transfer of a stable infant/child to lighting equivalent to the ICU, allowing proper physical assessment of the patient's colour and perfusion.

Loading

As transport trolleys of all kinds are very heavy (> 150 kg), lifting transport systems in and out of ambulances should be avoided as this has substantial health and safety implications. There are two main safe loading options:

- A ramp with an electric winch. The ramp should be secure and long enough to avoid a steep climb
- A lift mounted at the tailgate of the ambulance.

Trolley/incubator interfaces with vehicle

There are two further areas where the interface between the transport trolley and the vehicle requires consideration—restraint and gas supply.

Restraint

It is essential for the safety of staff and patients that trolleys of all kinds are secured effectively in the vehicle. As a crash involving a neonatal transport team in the Northern Region in the early 1990s illustrated, traditional trolley restraints ("York" type) are inadequate.

For this reason it is essential that transport teams liaise with their vehicle provider to ensure that the safest restraints possible are provided. Following publication of the European stretcher standard, discussed above, ambulance services have made great progress in attending to trolley security. A number of devices and options are available, including trolley designs that are stable in crashes and additional security from extra devices, such as floor clamps to anchor the trolley via strapping to specially strengthened slots in the floor.

All other devices such as monitors, pumps, and ventilators should also be secured. Restraining bolts and cargo straps are both good options. Do not carry unrestrained "extras".

All of these devices are only as good as the people using them on each transfer, and teams must be aware of the standard of restraint that is required and not depart on a transfer until this is achieved.

Gas supply

All emergency ambulances will carry an oxygen supply that must be secured within the ambulance. The team need to check the ambulance supply of oxygen is sufficient for their journey. Oxygen supply from the ambulance should be used during transport to conserve the transport incubator or trolley supply. Transport personnel should be familiar with vehicle gas supplies, so that they can monitor cylinder contents and ensure continuity of supply.

If a compressed air cylinder supply is needed this must also be secured and extra cylinders should not be taken into ambulances that are not secured. Further gas supply issues are discussed in chapter 4.

Speed and safety

There are two key components to safety: restraint and speed. Restraint is discussed above, but it should be remembered that restraining devices will all fail if challenged by a combination of heavy equipment and high speed collision. This is why the European standard for transport incubator systems limits the weight of the equipment.

Speed, and in particular the use of lights and sirens, needs careful consideration. A study by Auerbach in the USA looked at ambulances that were involved in road traffic accidents, and examined key features of each crash. It found that when ambulances were running with lights and sirens, any accident was more likely to yield an injured victim. Accidents happened most often at intersections, and so the most common incident was a side-on collision. These were not trivial accidents—two people were killed and another 18 sustained injuries classified as moderate or severe. Seat-belts were found to be protective for passengers and the authors concluded that to "maximise safety … passenger restraints be worn … speed limits obeyed if at all possible and all traffic signals heeded at intersections".

Another study, by Hunt, looked at the time saved by using lights and sirens in an urban setting. By comparing real emergency runs from accident scenes to hospital with journeys over the same route undertaken at normal traffic speed, the author was able to conclude that the time saved, an average of 43 seconds, was "… not clinically significant, except in rare circumstances". While most neonatal and paediatric transfers in the UK are over substantially longer distances than this, we have no comparable data on the time savings that might be expected or the clinical benefits of the time saved. An important principle from this study is that if traffic is moving normally use of lights and sirens does not result in substantial time savings.

The decision to use lights and sirens on a transfer is, therefore, a serious one. The default position should be that the ambulance will proceed at normal traffic speed and any other decision should be made by the transport team with the help of the ambulance crew, after considering these questions.

- Are the traffic conditions such that lights and sirens will facilitate a substantial improvement in journey time?

- Is the condition of the patient such that the scale of the shortening of the journey will be clinically significant?

These clinical indicators are the only justification for lights and sirens.

Other simpler and safer methods may yield more substantial time savings, for example by avoiding getting lost by keeping a set of maps that is up to date and written directions to hospitals visited. Some ambulances have a satellite navigation system to help guide them, or they can request the local ambulance service to help direct them to their destination. This will vary from region to region and should be negotiated by the ambulance personnel.

Patient safety

First and foremost, keep the staff safe so that they can help the patient.

Restraint for neonatal patients in incubators is an unresolved problem. No system is available that will reliably restrain a sick neonate in the event of a crash. There are substantial design problems in producing a system that will improve safety while allowing intensive care to proceed and without stripping the skin. This is an issue which clearly needs some clarity and evidence-based practice to ensure that infants are safely secured during transport.

Children transported on a trolley can be secured with a child-restraining mattress (Paedimate; Ferno, Bradford, UK). These are suitable for large infants and children up to 4 years, and effectively strap the child to the trolley using a five-point harness. Older children may be secured using two lap belts attached to the trolley.

> Safety in transit is promoted by:
> - Limiting the weight of trolley/incubator systems
> - Using restraining devices that are approved for the purpose
> - Limiting the use of lights and sirens to situations where any time saved will be clinically significant.

Ambulance crew and liaison with the ambulance service

Ambulance crews for transfers

Specialist transport-trained intensive care staff attend most UK paediatric and neonatal transfers.

A highly skilled paramedic ambulance crew is therefore not always necessary. An ambulance crew that are trained in emergency driving, should this be needed, are essential. The crew need to be clear about where the team need to go, and how urgently they need to arrive at the destination. Once the team have assessed the infant/child at the referring hospital, it would be helpful to give the crew an indication of how long the team expect to take stabilising the infant/child. This may be an opportunity for the ambulance crew to refuel for the return journey.

Dedicated vehicles

Dedicated vehicles are ambulances that are not part of the wider A&E fleet and are specially configured for interhospital transfer. They may be dedicated for use by one unit or hospital, or shared by several. Some units have experimented with operating the vehicle themselves, without the ambulance service, though this is not common. There are some advantages and disadvantages of the dedicated vehicle system compared to one where the transport team can use any frontline ambulance.

> *Advantages:*
> The vehicle may be optimally configured for restraining the transport trolley.
> Gas supplies can be increased and configured for team needs.
> Power supply to transport equipment may be optimised.
> Clinical supplies may be stored on the vehicle.
> The environment can be optimised for providing mobile intensive care.
> Where the frontline ambulance service is struggling to meet response targets, there may be benefits for both ICU and ambulance service in organising retrieval services separately.
>
> *Disadvantages:*
> If this becomes the only vehicle the team can use, there will be a problem mounting a transfer when the vehicle is being serviced, is broken down, or is being used by another team.
> Without a dedicated crew, there may be delays initiating transfer while a crew from another vehicle is diverted to pick up the dedicated vehicle.
> Long term replacement may be an issue when the vehicle becomes old and unreliable.

Planning with the ambulance service

It is helpful to have regular contact with senior personnel at the ambulance service, perhaps at an occasional meeting to discuss mutually important issues. Ambulance services are quite rightly focused on achieving high standards in their core activities relating to 999 calls. A similar commitment to interhospital transfers can be achieved when both transport teams and ambulance services recognise and respect each other's workload and priorities.

Staff comfort

Staff should appreciate the difficulty of performing any operation while the ambulance is moving, due to acceleration/deceleration and lateral movement. If an intervention is needed, the ambulance should be stopped before it is undertaken.

Riding in the back of an ambulance can cause motion sickness, even to the hardiest traveller. This is exacerbated by the type of suspension the ambulance has, by uneven bumpy roads, by travelling seated sideways, and by the inability to see out of the ambulance and obtain appropriate visual fixation. Tiredness, stress, hunger, and anxiety also exacerbate motion sickness. Various treatments for motion sickness are available, and transport staff who are afflicted may try to find one that suits, without causing drowsiness. Retrievals may take many hours to complete. It is advisable to take along a snack and drink for each member of the team.

Summary
Ambulance services and transport teams should cooperate to provide safe effective vehicles for transport. Particular attention should be given to planning for effective restraining devices for equipment and staff.
The ambulance environment is not ideal for intensive care. Remember that supplies of gas, power, and clinical equipment are all limited, so ensure they are used effectively.
Lights and sirens should only be used when clinically indicated.

4 Equipment and monitoring

Objectives
Be aware of transport-specific equipment.
Know limitations of transport equipment.
Assess level of monitoring required for transport.
Be able to evaluate the utility for transport of items
    of equipment.

Introduction

Transport equipment should be complete and adequate for the provision of continuous intensive care throughout the transport episode. Equipment must be specific to transport and maintained by the transport team. All staff should be trained in the use of the transport equipment and must be familiar with its whereabouts for ease of access. Transport staff should regularly check the equipment and be able to troubleshoot equipment and monitoring problems. It is a paediatric intensive care (PIC) standard, and good practice generally, that the retrieval team has annual updates to include equipment training.

Equipment should be sufficient to provide the required level of intensive care, but should not be so comprehensive as to cause risks with the sheer volume carried. Consideration should be given to the amount of equipment stored on an ambulance as most ambulance chassis have a maximum gross vehicle weight of 3·5–4·6 tonne.

The market for specialist transport equipment is low volume with a limited number of suppliers. For this reason it tends to be relatively expensive and slow to evolve.

General features of all equipment

Key characteristics

- Self-contained, lightweight, and portable
- Be durable and robust to withstand repeated use
- Long battery life and short recharge time
- Clear displays
- Suitable for all ages transferred
- Visible and audible alarms
- Data storage and download capability
- Secure

The British Paediatric Association, the British Paediatric Intensive Care Society, and the American Academy of Pediatrics have drawn up guidelines on transport equipment. When selecting equipment one should be sure to meet these guidelines.

Equipment that is built for transport is preferable to general intensive care unit (ICU) equipment, which may be less reliable and robust.

Electrical components should run off mains power, have an internal battery, and be able to take power from the vehicle.

Trolleys

To be conveyed in an ambulance the equipment needs to be on a trolley, and a number of options are available.

Neonatal transport teams have the advantage of very small patients, so there is room on a trolley for the infant and all the necessary equipment. Without exception ground transfer neonatal teams use an adapted ambulance trolley for this purpose, the precise trolley choice being determined by the local ambulance service.

Some paediatric transport teams utilise the ambulance's own stretcher trolley and secure equipment to it once they are in the vehicle. Others have adapted conventional ambulance trolleys.

Paediatric transfer trolleys need space to accommodate an older child with adequate restraining straps, a multichannel monitor, a transport ventilator and oxygen supply, and space for six infusion devices. Ideally this equipment should be placed below the patient to minimise risk to the patient, should the vehicle be involved in a sudden brake or impact.

For all trolleys the key feature is security and restraint in the vehicle in the event of a crash, and this is discussed in chapter 3.

Batteries

Most electrical items of transport equipment have internal rechargeable batteries. Although in theory these batteries last for several hours, long enough for most transports, in practice they are not so straightforward.

Rechargeable batteries need routine maintenance to keep them working effectively. Merely leaving an item of equipment plugged in and "charging" for several weeks is not enough. Rechargeable batteries need to be regularly completely drained and then fully recharged in order to remain efficient.

Figure 4.1 illustrates an effective battery maintenance and use cycle, including planned battery discharge. Figure 4.2 illustrates a cycle of battery use and charging that results in the battery becoming less effective.

For this reason it is necessary for batteries to be properly maintained. Even with good planned maintenance procedures, rechargeable batteries will need replacing occasionally, approximately once a year.

On transport, always use external sources of power when these are available. If possible, choose equipment that is not solely reliant on internal rechargeable batteries. The options are either that the device may be run from the ambulance power or that the batteries are accessible and may be replaced in the event of failure.

> Look after your batteries—do not rely on leaving them charging all the time and hoping for the best.

Ventilators

A transport ventilator must be portable, light, robust, and easy to operate. Disconnection and high pressure alarms are essential. Most transport ventilators are gas driven, meaning they need only a gas supply, not electricity, to work. Ventilators with complex electrical systems are unlikely to work properly in transit. Any ventilator which stops working in the event of a power failure is highly undesirable for transport.

Gas driven ventilators may consume 8·5–20 litres per min, or more, of gas and this needs to be remembered when calculating the oxygen requirements for the journey. Some ventilators have facilities that reduce compressed gas consumption. A particularly useful one is the ability to entrain air from the environment to blend with compressed oxygen.

Positive end expiratory pressure (PEEP) may be added to continuous flow ventilators without this facility by adding a PEEP valve to the circuit.

The delivered oxygen concentration should be monitored with a fuel cell oxygen analyser and should be variable from 21 to 100%.

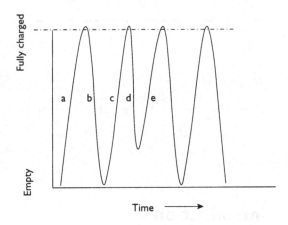

Figure 4.1 a = Battery is charged to full. b = Fully discharged to empty in a planned maintenance episode. c = Fully charged again. d = Taken on a transfer and partially drained. e = Fully charged again. Process continues.

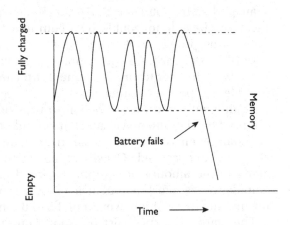

Figure 4.2 A less effective charging process. Here the battery is repeatedly charged to full and then taken on transfers that partially drain it. Over many such cycles the battery develops a "memory" of the lowest level it is discharged to, and "forgets" that it can be discharged even further. When the team goes on a longer transfer, the battery fails even though it might have been expected to last longer.

A ventilator appropriate to the size of the child should be available for all transfers, as well as a hand-bagging system for emergencies. In general, neonatal patients need a pressure limited, time cycled ventilator while paediatric patients will need a volume control facility. Some paediatric transport teams carry two ventilators to accommodate the wide specification required.

Gas supply

Compressed gases are very precious transport resources. Most transfers need a compressed oxygen source, and some will also need compressed air.

The importance of carrying sufficient gas, and being careful in its use during transport, cannot be stressed too highly. Ensure the ambulance supply is compatible with the transport equipment and adequate for the journey time. You should have sufficient gas available for double the expected length of the journey to allow for unforeseen circumstances. There should be a sufficient supply on the incubator/trolley to cover the transfer to and from the ambulance. Appendix 2 gives formulae for calculating how many litres of gas may be needed on a transfer and how many minutes of gas supply are in a cylinder.

Printed on the neck of all gas cylinders is important information about their contents when full. The standard "F" cylinder has a "bull nose" valve type and holds 1360 litres, and an "E" cylinder has a pin index valve and contains 680 litres. Cylinders carried in most ambulances today are classified "HX" and have a star valve. They contain 2300 litres and there may be two of them. The pressure the cylinder has been filled to is displayed on a gauge. Cylinders should always be full for transfer and checked regularly.

Under no circumstances should additional gas cylinders be placed insecurely in ambulances. Great care and respect should be given to pressurised gas cylinders, as they are potentially lethal in an accident.

Oxygen supply

Oxygen is usually delivered from cylinders, but liquid oxygen is used by some specialised services. This has the advantage of being a relatively large supply, but it is expensive and training is required in its use and maintenance.

Air supply

Air may be delivered from three sources.

1. The atmosphere. Some ventilators can entrain atmospheric air and blend this with a compressed oxygen supply. The compressed oxygen is needed to drive the ventilator, but the air can be blended with the oxygen to achieve inspired oxygen concentrations (Fio_2)

from 0·4 to 1·0. At Fio_2 around 0·5, this is a very gas efficient mode.

2. Cylinders, as for oxygen. In general ambulances do not carry air cylinders and this can make air a relatively precious gas. Arrangements may be made to install extra secured air cylinders in the vehicle when required.

3. Compressor. Some neonatal transport trolley systems may be supplied with a compressor which provides a compressed air supply to the ventilator using atmospheric air. Compressors have the advantage over cylinders of not running out, but the disadvantage that if they suffer an electrical failure they don't work.

> Gas is precious—conserve it at all times by using external supplies. Monitor cylinder contents frequently in transit to avoid unexpected failure.

Humidification

Humidification of inspired gases is important to reduce the risk of partial or complete endotracheal tube blockage by dried secretions. This is particularly so in infants, who have narrower endotracheal tubes than adults or older children, and on long transfers. The use of poorly humidified gases also worsens lung injury, promotes sputum retention and may lead to atelectasis. Adequate humidification may be achieved by using disposable heat and moisture exchangers (HMEs) of an appropriate size for the patient, or by using portable heated water humidifiers. HMEs are simple, lightweight and do not require any external power, so are not prone to failure. Although they increase the resistance and the dead space of the ventilator circuit, this does not appear to be a problem in clinical practice, even with very small premature babies.

Heated water humidifiers use considerable power and are technically difficult to use in a moving environment, due to the water sloshing around.

Temperature maintenance

Heat loss occurs by four main mechanisms, and each is accentuated as patient size is reduced.

1. By *radiation* to cooler surrounding objects such as ambulance walls and windows. Ambulances are rarely insulated, and so this

must be reduced by reducing skin exposure or placing infants in an incubator. Infants may also lose heat rapidly when moving from the warm ward to the ambulance outside the hospital, often with its doors open and a wind blowing through it. When you are nearly ready to leave the referring hospital, it is sensible to ask one of the ambulance crew to go back to the ambulance, shut the doors and run the engine with the heating full on to warm the ambulance up prior to loading the child.

2. By *conduction* directly from the patient to cold objects placed in contact, such as cold blankets. Transport incubators and blankets should be prewarmed before use.

3. By *convection* when cool air flows across the child, for instance when incubator portholes are open, or when the ambulance doors are opened.

4. By *evaporation* either from the skin, especially in very premature neonates, or from the respiratory tract.

Infants, especially small preterm infants, are particularly at risk of excessive heat loss. A large surface to volume ratio, less adipose insulation, an inability to change posture to reduce heat loss, and smaller amounts of brown fat tissue compared to more mature infants all mean that the infant will react less well to cold stress. In addition, brown fat metabolism in response to cold increases oxygen demands and may worsen hypoxia. The *neutral thermal environment* is the temperature range within which a minimal amount of energy is used by the babies to maintain their body temperature.

Incubators

Incubators should be used for transporting small (< 5 kg) or premature infants. The incubator should allow good visibility, easy access to the child, a constant ambient temperature, and stable inspired oxygen concentration.

Access to the patient differs between models of incubators. For routine procedures, access via portholes on both sides of the incubator is helpful. For emergency procedures, such as intubation, the patient tray should slide out. A tray that slides out of the head end of the incubator is useful in this situation, allowing airway control and intubation without exposing the whole baby. A heating system that is fan

assisted may also be better at retaining heat in a clinical emergency.

An incubator that supports environmental humidity may be preferable for very immature babies. Systems that use a water-soaked sponge are surprisingly effective, yielding 80–90% humidity after an hour or so of operation, and their simplicity means there is nothing to go wrong.

Babies receiving complex intensive care need good access for copious tubes and lines into the incubator.

Incubators have a relatively large power consumption and so rely on an additional battery supply within the unit.

Suggested initial incubator temperature settings for neonates. This is just a guide, and the infant's current temperature, current incubator temperature and size all need to be taken into account.

Weight	Initial temperature setting (°C)
> 2500 g	33
1500–2500 g	35
1000–1500 g	36
< 1000 g	39

Incubators allow the infant to be left unclothed to observe chest movement and skin colour. A blanket or reflective cover over the incubator will reduce heat loss further, but will also prevent observation of the child.

Other warming equipment

Chemical warming mattresses and blankets, such as Transwarmer (Advanced Health Technologies, Herts, UK), may be used to help maintain body temperature for several hours. They may be used as an additional warming method for an infant in a transport incubator or for a child on a transport trolley. This method of warming is not controllable and care needs to be taken as these mattresses can get very hot (temperatures of 40°C). A sheet should be placed between the mattress and the skin, particularly for premature infants, and continuous temperature monitoring observed.

Containers or surgical gloves filled with hot water should not be used to warm an infant or child as they may spill or burst, leading to scalds.

This section has concentrated on heat loss, as this is by far the commonest situation. Hyperthermia can occur when larger babies are in incubators on rare occasions when the sun is shining brightly through onto the incubator, which acts like a greenhouse. Avoid bright sunlight on incubators.

Pyrexia should also be controlled by proper use of antipyretic medications and the use of appropriate clothing or coverings. Take care that extremities do not get cold, as the child may start to shiver, which will then increase the central temperature.

Suction equipment

Portable suction must be provided in transport. Some devices use compressed gas from cylinders to generate suction, utilising the Venturi effect. These are simple and reliable devices, but they use lots of gas, particularly if continuous suction is needed. Care must be taken to account for this when calculating oxygen requirements.

Portable suction units which rely on battery power have the advantage of not using valuable compressed gas, but may be prone to battery failure unless run off the ambulance power.

Ambulances carry portable suction units, but as these are not as sophisticated as piped suction units available within the hospital environment, suction should be performed before leaving the referring hospital.

There are also foot pump units available which may be difficult to use in transit.

All of these suction devices provide suction that is intended for clearing the airway. This is relatively crude suction, applied for a brief period. There are two situations where low level continuous suction would be normal practice, and this is problematical for transport where the suction devices are much too powerful.

1. Infants with oesophageal atresia with a replogle tube in the oesophageal pouch. Normal practice on the NICU is to leave the tube on continuous low level suction to keep the pouch drained of secretions and avoid aspiration. Continuous high level suction can traumatise the oesophageal pouch and impede surgical repair. The simplest solution for transfer is to suction the tube intermittently, but frequently, either with a syringe or by leaving it attached to the suction device and turning it on for a few seconds every 5–10 minutes, ensuring the secretions have been cleared each time.
2. Some pneumothoraces continually recollect, particularly in ventilated patients, and low level suction is needed on the chest drain to

keep the lung expanded. Continuous high level suction can traumatise the lung. In the first instance, try the infant without suction. Just because the infant needed suction a few hours ago does not mean he or she still does. If the infant does not tolerate withdrawal of suction then it will be necessary to provide continuous low level suction. This may be achieved by connecting the chest drain circuit to transport suction in the normal way, but with a break or hole in the circuit to attenuate the suction. This is most elegantly achieved with a Y-connector, but a hole in the tubing suffices.

Be aware that suction may be labelled in various units (kPa, bar or mmHg).

Infusion pumps

Gravity driven drips and infusion devices that measure drip rates are affected by movement and therefore not reliable in transport. For neonatal and paediatric transport syringe pump devices are used. These allow accurate delivery of small volumes of fluid/medication to infants and children.

> *Infusion pumps:*
> Should be able to accurately deliver flow rates from 0·1 ml/h
> Should be able to bolus dose
> Should have occlusion, excess pressure, infusion complete, syringe disengaged and low battery alarms
> Should be light, compact, and robust
> Should be easy to use
> Should have long battery life.

At least six should be carried on paediatric transfers, as this is the PIC standard. At least three are needed on neonatal transfers, with up to six available as required for more complex transfers.

The biggest problem with infusion pumps in transport practice is their short battery life. Some syringe pumps are powered by standard alkaline batteries that may be changed by the transport team if they fail. Another good solution is to designate pumps for transport and change the batteries often.

Defibrillators

A defibrillator is not needed on neonatal transfers, except in rare cases of shockable arrhythmia. A portable defibrillator should be carried by paediatric teams, ensuring "intensive care on the move". Although used rarely in children, staff need to be familiar with their use.

Paramedic ambulances will have a defibrillator on board. These may be of the automatic external defibrillator (AED) type, as recommended for children over 8 years of age. The transport team need to be familiar with the type of defibrillator available.

When using a defibrillator, it is the current flowing across the myocardium that is effective. This is maximised by a number of factors.

- The energy selected. Many defibrillators default to 200 J as the first energy setting. This should be adjusted to the appropriate energy level based on the weight of the child.
- The electrode position (Fig. 4.3). Either just to the right of the upper part of the sternum and in the fifth intercostal space in the midclavicular line, or anteroposterior, i.e. over the left shoulder blade and in the fourth intercostal space in the midclavicular line. The latter position is useful in young children and infants.
- The electrode polarity is not critical, although one is normally marked "Sternum" and one "Apex".
- Paddle size. Should be the largest that will make contact with the chest, taking care to make sure that the paddles do not touch.
- The use of gel pads and firm pressure improve the passage of energy from the paddles to the patient, and reduce the risks of burns. KY Jelly and wet pads are not adequate and may lead to burns. Alcoholic tinctures may ignite, and oxygen may explode.

Caution. Defibrillators deliver serious amounts of energy to the patient *and anyone else in electrical contact with the patient.* Before defibrillating, it is your responsibility to make sure that everyone is clear, including yourself. Merely shouting "Charging to 200" in the style of *ER* is not enough.

Hands-free paddles are probably safer for transport use.

> Select equipment carefully for transport and be familiar with the features and limitations of the equipment available.

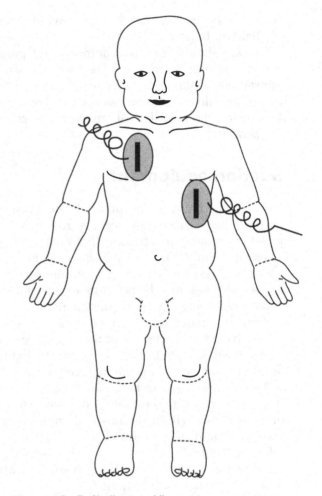

Figure 4.3 Defibrillator paddle positions.

Monitoring

Monitoring critically ill patients during transport is essential to detect changes in their condition in an environment where observation and auscultation are much more difficult. The proper monitoring of vital signs will allow detection of early signs of patient deterioration and the ability to respond to these before they become critical. It may be difficult to assess how much or how little monitoring a patient requires. Very sick or unstable children will require extensive monitoring, whilst those who are stable may require less. Accurate assessment of the child is therefore important. The possibility of monitoring the following parameters during transport is essential.

- Heart rate/ECG
- Respiratory rate
- Oxygen saturation
- 2 × invasive pressure monitoring
- Non-invasive blood pressure
- 2 × temperature
- End tidal CO_2 (paediatrics)

Monitors—features and clinical applications

Monitors should meet the general criteria for transport equipment, given above. They should monitor all the desired parameters. A data storage and download capability may be useful. At present simple two-colour screens are preferable to multicoloured monitors as they have longer battery life.

Monitoring heart rate

The ECG monitor is used to detect electrical activity of the cardiac muscles using pregelled electrodes as sensors, an amplifier, and a device to record it (Fig. 4.4).

Movement of the child clearly cannot be avoided during transport, and this may cause interference and a poor quality ECG trace. Artefacts such as those caused by movement can be eliminated by optimising the ECG recording technique.

Avoid artefacts by:
Cleaning the skin
Drying the skin to ensure good adhesion
Storing the pregelled electrodes properly to avoid them drying out
Only using the electrodes once
Ensuring that the lead clips and any other connections fit snugly
Placing the electrodes on bony prominences to reduce skin and muscle movement
Placing the electrodes in the correct positions, as shown in Fig. 4.4
Filtering the ECG
Adjusting the gain to optimise the size of the ECG complexes
Setting the alarms 10–15 beats above and below the heart rate
Keeping the child warm, as shivering will produce artefacts.

Respiratory monitoring

Generally the size of the respiratory waveform equates to the depth of the child's respiration.

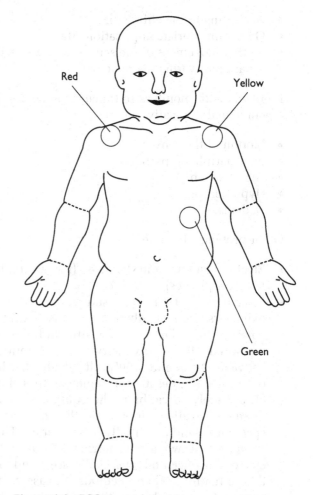

Figure 4.4 ECG electrode positions.

However, even an obstructed airway can show some respiratory trace, and therefore clinical assessment is vital.

It is important to:

- Set appropriate alarm limits for the age of the patient
- Set the alarms to detect apnoea as well as respiratory rate
- Clinically assess respiration regularly by observing chest movement
- Remember that the commonest cause for a drop in heart rate is inadequate ventilation.

Oxygen saturation monitoring

Saturation monitoring is only accurate if the sensor is applied properly:

- According to the child's size
- On an appropriate application site
- So that movement of the sensor is minimised
- If dark nail varnish is removed.

Problems with monitors in transport arise due to a poor signal, typically due to:

- Motion of the sensor
- Poor peripheral perfusion
- Hypotension
- Hypothermia
- Oedema.

Other problems include:

- Electromagnetic interference (for example, from cellphones)
- Inaccuracy at lower saturations. Pulse oximeters are calibrated against values obtained from the blood of healthy individuals measured by co-oximetry at saturations between 80% and 100%. It would hardly be ethical to desaturate someone to below 80% merely to calibrate the equipment, and therefore readings less than this are more speculative and potentially less accurate. This is important when transferring infants with cyanotic congenital heart disease, and in this situation other methods of assessing oxygenation, such as transcutaneous P_{O_2} monitoring, may be preferred
- Probe position—be aware that pre- and postductal saturations may differ substantially in infants with a significant ductal shunt
- Response delay. Many pulse oximeters use averaging techniques over a number of beats to give a more reliable value. This means that the technique gives a relatively late warning of desaturation. For this reason there should be separate ventilation and disconnect alarms in the transport system
- Equally there may be a delay in recovery of the oxygen saturation after effective ventilation is re-established
- Bright lights can overload the sensor and lead to an inaccurate reading
- Carboxyhaemoglobinaemia makes the oximeter overread, lulling the attendants into a false sense of security. Pulse oximetry must not be relied upon in a patient who is at risk of carbon monoxide poisoning
- Methaemoglobinaemia also affects pulse oximetry, causing the device to underread

- Pulsatile veins may confuse the pulse oximeter and lead to an inaccurate measurement.

Be suspicious of a reading of around 85%, especially with a poor waveform, or where it does not correlate with the patient's condition. A detected ratio of red : infrared light of one gives a saturation of 85% with many pulse oximeters, and this reading can be obtained by taking the oximeter probe off the patient and waving it rhythmically in the air!

Transcutaneous blood gas monitoring

This technique is widely used in the NICU where the relatively thin and immature skin of the neonate improves the reliability of the readings. Both transcutaneous oxygen (TcP_{O_2}) and carbon dioxide (TcP_{CO_2}) may be measured. This technique may also be applied in transport, as the monitors (TINA, Radiometer, Copenhagen, Denmark) are fairly small and have a good external battery facility. A randomised trial, by O'Connor, of using these monitors in transported ventilated neonates found that infants transferred with TcP_{CO_2} monitoring completed the transfer with significantly better blood gases and had their ventilation settings reduced, compared to infants transferred without the monitoring.

To set the monitor up on an infant being transferred:

- Warm the monitor up while the infant is being stabilised
- After transfer into the transport incubator apply the probe to the baby, and allow the readings to stabilise (5–10 minutes)
- Do a blood gas and follow the procedure for calibrating the monitor to the gas results. If only capillary blood gas is available, calibrate just the TcP_{CO_2}
- Make any adjustments to the treatment regimen necessary on the basis of the blood gas, and depart on the transfer.

Use the readings on the transcutaneous monitor to keep blood gases within the desired range. This is a generally reliable technique. In transit be aware that bizarre or wildly fluctuating readings probably indicate the probe is losing contact with the skin. In shocked infants with poor skin perfusion the system is less reliable.

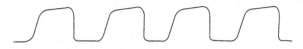

Figure 4.5 Typical capnograph.

End tidal CO₂ monitoring

End tidal CO_2 monitoring (ET_{CO_2} or capnography) is the graphic record of instantaneous CO_2 concentration in the respired gases during a respiratory cycle (Fig. 4.5). It indicates changes in the elimination of CO_2 from the lungs, and indirectly reflects changes in CO_2 levels in the blood. However, the exact relationship between ET_{CO_2} and Pa_{CO_2} in critically ill children is not always clear, as ET_{CO_2} is affected by details of pulmonary blood flow and alveolar ventilation, as well as the Pa_{CO_2}. Nevertheless, capnography provides a useful trend, gives information about the pattern of respiration, and acts as an extra ventilator disconnect alarm.

ET_{CO_2} monitoring is considered mandatory for patients intubated and ventilated for anaesthesia, and is frequently used in the PICU. Given that the aim of a retrieval service is to provide mobile intensive care, ET_{CO_2} monitoring should be undertaken in ventilated children during transport.

The technique is not widely used in the NICU, where studies have failed to demonstrate utility. To monitor mainstream ET_{CO_2} requires introducing a probe into the ventilator circuit, which may be significant in extending the dead space of the tubing in the neonate. Its use in transport of neonates may be a topic for further investigation.

Inspired oxygen concentration monitoring

Oxygen analysers are needed for ambient oxygen therapy as well as in ventilator circuits. Some transport incubators have an oxygen analyser incorporated within the transport system. Oxygen concentration alarms may be useful.

Blood gas monitoring

New technology allows portable blood gas monitoring in transit. These devices have not been fully evaluated for paediatric or neonatal transport. They may have a valuable role on long journeys, but most ventilated patients should have a blood gas analysis prior to leaving the referring hospital and then be managed on the transport monitoring for the journey.

Non-invasive blood pressure monitoring

This should be available for all transported children, although it is fraught with difficulties in practice. Measurement by auscultation is often impossible and measurement by palpation is inaccurate and may be misleading. Automated non-invasive blood pressure monitoring measurements are affected by vibration and motion. All non-invasive methods tend to overestimate low blood pressure and underestimate high blood pressure. However, they may give reasonable indication of blood pressure trend.

Frequent non-invasive blood pressure monitoring consumes a lot of power, and will deplete the monitor battery quickly.

Cuffs of different sizes should be carried. The appropriate size cuff will cover two-thirds of the upper arm, and the balloon should almost encircle the arm. Too small a cuff overestimates blood pressure.

Invasive pressure monitoring

Invasive blood pressure monitoring is more reliable than non-invasive methods in the haemodynamically unstable child, and should be considered in any child who is shocked, requiring large volumes of fluids, or receiving inotropic support.

The pressure monitoring system consists of an indwelling catheter, tubing, transducer, and monitor. The tubing is filled with saline or heparinised saline and attached to a thin diaphragm. This converts changes in pressure and mechanical energy into an electrical signal which is displayed as a waveform on the monitor.

The system is calibrated to provide accurate measurement by opening the stopcock to air, thereby creating a zero baseline. From this baseline, positive and negative changes can be detected. The transducer should be placed at the level of the chest, and in the event of sudden, unexplained changes in the measured pressure, the transducer position should be checked to ensure that it hasn't fallen to the floor.

There are advantages and disadvantages in invasive pressure monitoring.

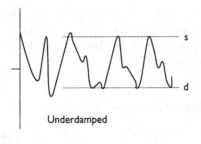

Underdamped

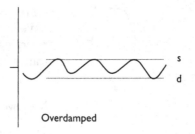

Overdamped

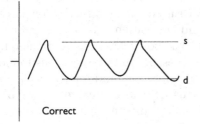

Correct

Figure 4.6 Damping of the arterial trace. s = systolic pressure, d = diastolic pressure.

Advantages
Accurate
Can be used for blood sampling and blood gases
Waveform may be analysed
May be used to count the heart rate—is less prone to motion artefact than ECG monitoring

Disadvantages
Risk of haemorrhage
May be affected by motion
Invasive catheter placement needed, with consequent risk of distal hypoperfusion

Inadequate damping, overdamping, or movement artefact may affect the measured systolic and diastolic pressures (Fig. 4.6), and in these circumstances the mean pressure will be more reliable.

Temperature monitoring

Continuous monitoring of temperature is essential to regulate incubator temperature for neonates and environmental temperature for children transported on trolleys. Central and peripheral temperature should be measured in small infants and children who are shocked or unstable.

Most transport monitors have the facility to monitor central and peripheral temperatures.

Central temperature in neonates may be measured by lightly securing a probe in the axilla. Position the baby in the transport incubator slightly turned to one side. Use the lower axilla, ensuring the upper arm is by the side of the baby, keeping the temperature probe snug.

Nasopharyngeal and rectal probes are also used, particularly in older children, and the extra reliability of these may be important in very sick patients with skin hypoperfusion.

Temperature probes are affected by improper placement. For example, if they are placed too close to a large blood vessel or high flow organ such as the liver, they may read reassuringly high. Conversely, falsely low readings occur if the probe has poor contact with the skin, or in the presence of vasoconstriction. One of the commonest reasons for an acute fall in rectal temperature during transport is that the probe has fallen out.

Monitoring of core and peripheral temperature can be used as an indicator of shock, and should be assessed in conjunction with the other clinical signs outlined in this manual.

Blood glucose monitoring

Blood glucose should be routinely measured during the stabilisation phase in the referring hospital, and more often if there have been previous problems with glucose homoeostasis, in diabetics, newborn infants, patients on restricted fluids, and if insulin is being given.

A handheld glucometer should be part of the transport equipment.

Inspired nitric oxide concentration monitoring

There are few monitors available for transport use. The Printernox (Micro Medical) has a short battery life but may be adapted to use an additional battery supply, for example the external battery on the incubator transport system. It is desirable that NO and NO_2 are measured during delivery. This needs to be monitored near to the patient, after ensuring gas mixing.

Finally

Good planning, anticipation and knowing your equipment will ensure a safe transport; however, you may find yourself in a situation where the equipment fails you. For this reason, always make sure you can ventilate your patient—a

self-inflating Ambu-bag close at hand is essential. If an infusion pump fails, compromise a less vital infusion, one that can be administered by bolus. If your monitor fails try to utilise the ambulance equipment (some ambulances carry saturation monitors, as do the RAF Search and Rescue helicopters). If no monitoring is available utilise a stethoscope and basic assessment skills. The worst that can happen is that the ambulance will break down as well.

Summary
Planning and maintenance are necessary for transport equipment to be effective.
Awareness of the limitations of transport equipment is important in ensuring safe transport.
Well set-up monitoring is an excellent resource for clinical decision making in transit.
Know your kit.

5 Air transport of critically ill children

Introduction

The use of aircraft to transport sick children between hospitals can greatly reduce transport times compared to ground transportation. This is essential when large distances are involved, i.e. between countries. It may also prove useful when children are extremely ill and require transfer for specialist treatment such as neurosurgery or extracorporeal membrane oxygenation (ECMO). In this context air transport is indicated if the estimated ground transfer time exceeds two hours.

> *Objectives*
> To understand the advantages and disadvantages of air transport.
> To know the important safety aspects of air transport, particularly rotary wing transport.
> To highlight physiological problems specific to air transport and reduced barometric pressure.

Choice of aircraft

Both fixed wing and rotary wing aircraft (helicopters) may be used for aeromedical transport. However, once the flying time exceeds three hours then fixed wing aircraft are preferred.

Helicopters

These aircraft are usually unpressurised and relatively slow, 100 knots being the usual cruising speed for a Sea-King. Helicopters are faster than fixed wing aircraft for short journeys, because they are able to land near or at the hospitals at both ends. In general most journeys by air within the UK are quicker by helicopter because of their versatility in use of landing grounds. The lack of cabin pressurisation can be a problem when transporting extremely hypoxic patients as the reduction in oxygen pressure that occurs at altitude can be clinically significant in the patient with extreme respiratory failure. This problem can be circumvented by asking the pilot to fly low. In normal weather conditions military pilots will usually be happy to fly at 150 m which does not exacerbate hypoxia.

Many different aircraft are used to transport patients, and some have been specially outfitted as air ambulances.

Many of these aircraft are cramped and do not afford full access to the patient, especially the airway. Also many smaller civilian helicopters do not have the more sophisticated navigational, avionics, and night flying capability of military aircraft. Although military aircraft do not have customised air ambulance facilities this is offset by the rapid mobilisation, night flying capability, and size of the Sea-King. This allows good patient access.

Disadvantages of helicopters include the noise and vibration and, in winter, extreme cold. Even military helicopters will be unable to fly in dense fog or snow (as the pilot needs to see the ground to land). High winds may also preclude helicopter use.

Certain safety precautions are essential when using helicopters for aeromedical transport. These start by ensuring that the landing ground is approved for helicopter use. If an impromptu landing area is being used, i.e. if evacuating a casualty from an accident scene, it is helpful to station an emergency vehicle (police car/ambulance, etc.) at the windward side of the landing area. The vehicle should be positioned facing down wind, and should have its headlights and blue lights illuminated. This is especially important at night. The surrounding area must be cleared of bystanders and spectators, as the down draft from the helicopter can throw up debris and even blow people over. The presence of rubbish in or near the landing ground is an additional hazard that should be avoided. Foreign object damage (FOD) from something as seemingly innocuous as a polythene bag has caused enough damage to aircraft to precipitate a crash.

The transport team should wait 50–100 m from the edge of the landing ground and should stay there until the helicopter has landed. The loadmaster will usually then leave the aircraft and instruct the transport team how to proceed. Helicopters should only be approached from the front in order to avoid the tail rotor. Smaller helicopters also pose a hazard from the main

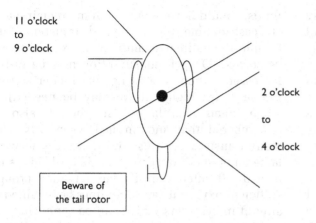

11 o'clock
to
9 o'clock

2 o'clock
to
4 o'clock

Beware of
the tail rotor

Figure 5.1 Safe approaches to the Sea-King.

rotor. However, in the Sea-King this is at a height of about 3 m, and so poses little threat (Fig. 5.1). This feature makes "hot loading" (i.e. with the rotors still rotating) relatively safe in the Sea-King. In fact the RAF prefer to hot load as it reduces the risks of engine malfunction attendant on shutting the engines down. It is usual also to have the fire brigade and ambulance service in attendance. This is obviously essential in the event of a fire or accident.

If the rotors and engines are to be shut down the helicopter must not be approached until the blades have come to rest and the loadmaster gives permission to approach. This is because there is a risk of the helicopter capsising during shutdown. For the same reason when the helicopter lands at the hospital from which the patient is being collected the transport team should remain strapped in until the rotors have come to a complete stop and the loadmaster gives permission to unstrap.

Approaching the helicopter
Do not go under the rotors until clearly beckoned (or thumbs up).
Usually the loadmaster (winchman) will come out to you.
The starboard (rear) cabin door is used for stretchers.
The port (front) door—which has steps—may be used for walking passengers.
Remember that the pilot is still "flying" the aircraft while still on the ground (unless the rotor has stopped).
NEVER go around the back of the helicopter— touching the tail rotor will kill you.
When ready (loadmaster's decision), with no loose articles, walk—don't run—to the door and load.

Fixed wing aircraft

These are used when transferring patients distances of over approximately 300 miles (500 km). They are limited by the need to take off and land at airports, but their greater airspeed and range make them preferable for long distance transfers. Fixed wing aircraft usually fly at a higher altitude than helicopters and cabins may therefore be pressurised. This will ameliorate the reduction in barometric pressure that occurs at altitude. A commercial airliner flying at an altitude of approximately 11 000 m will have a cabin pressure of around 565 mmHg, equivalent to an altitude of around 2500 m. Thus whilst the *partial pressure* of oxygen remains the same (21% of the total air pressure), the *actual alveolar oxygen pressure* is decreased in proportion with the reduction in total barometric pressure, i.e. 21% × 565 mmHg = 119 mmHg. This would be equivalent to breathing 16% oxygen at sea level, and obviously necessitates an increase in Fio$_2$ in the hypoxic patient.

In areas where long distance transfers are more usual (Australia, Scottish Highlands and Islands) ambulance services will have fixed wing air ambulances. However, charter and scheduled commercial aircraft may also be used. The RAF do not provide a fixed wing transport service as the Search and Rescue (SAR) squadrons do not have suitable fixed wing aircraft. The United States Air Force (USAF) have considerable experience of long distance aeromedical transport.

- Air transport is usually faster if the ground transfer time exceeds two hours.
- In the UK helicopters are usually the quickest type of aircraft to use.
- Helicopters should be approached from the front to keep clear of the tail rotor.
- Instructions from aircrew should be obeyed at all times.
- Fixed wing aircraft may be faster for transfers exceeding 300 miles (500 km).

Equipment and supplies

During ground transport it is possible to stop the ambulance. This can allow further supplies of oxygen or drugs to be commandeered from a hospital en route. It also provides a quiet and stable environment for diagnosis and therapeutic intervention. This is rarely possible during air transport. It is therefore doubly necessary to ensure that enough equipment is carried to cope with any eventuality. Equipment should be appropriate for the age of the child and arranged in easily accessible bags. It is often helpful to think of and store items using an ABC (Airway, Breathing, Circulation) framework.

Another important factor that must be considered during air transport is radiofrequency interference (RFI). All electronic devices generate radio waves which can interfere with the function of other electronic devices nearby. Medical devices can also produce RFI. The USAF and RAF have a strict protocol for testing devices for RFI before they are used in the air. Many devices are certified by the US Federal Aviation Authority (FAA) as safe for aeromedical use, and should not produce RFI. It is also theoretically possible that RFI could be generated by the aircraft's equipment and cause the medical equipment to malfunction, although we are not aware of any reported instances of this.

Communication with base can be very difficult. Mobile phones cannot be used in the aircraft, but it may be possible to get a message to base hospital via the pilot. Two-way conversations are impossible, so if advice is needed it is preferable to seek this before take off.

- Take plenty of oxygen.
- Ensure electronic equipment does not cause radiofrequency interference.

General issues

The vibration encountered during helicopter transport can cause displacement of endotracheal tubes and intravascular lines. These must therefore be secured before take off. Usually the application of additional tape (Sleek) is effective in securing these devices. It is prudent to establish central venous access in all but the most stable patient, as peripheral IV lines often cease functioning at the most inopportune moment. If the patient is receiving inotropes, prostaglandin infusions, or magnesium, then central access is mandatory.

In any patient who is ill enough to warrant air transport an indwelling arterial line is also mandatory to allow accurate haemodynamic monitoring, and sampling for blood glucose measurement. It is also sensible to have non-invasive blood pressure monitoring available in the event of arterial line failure.

Cardiac arrest drugs and volume (i.e. human albumin solution 4·5%) appropriate for the patient's weight should be drawn up ready for use. Intravenous infusions, including maintenance

fluids, should have enough volume remaining for at least double the estimated transport time. Double the estimated amount of oxygen should be carried. Oxygen consumption may be further increased when operating at higher airway pressures (as higher flows may be needed), or when hand ventilating. It should also be remembered that suction is oxygen driven on many transport systems, and that this can waste large amounts of oxygen, especially if this is not turned off after use. If one has not brought sufficient oxygen it can sometimes be obtained on aircraft in cylinders which can be connected into a Waters circuit to allow hand ventilation. However, this facility should not be relied on.

Many authors prefer nasotracheal intubation for air transport. There is no doubt that it is easier to secure a nasal tube to the patient's face but one should not be lulled into a false sense of security, as the tracheal end of the tube can still move several centimetres if the head is moved. The head, and indeed the entire patient, should be secured inside the incubator/transport system so that movement is impossible. Vacuum mattresses, restraining straps and tape can be used to secure the patient. The ventilator circuit must be supported and strapped so that it does not move in relation to the patient's head. Ventilated patients should usually be fully sedated and paralysed to reduce the risk of inadvertent extubation, and in order to optimise their ventilation and haemodynamics.

It is impossible to hear anything with a stethoscope in any kind of aircraft. This makes diagnosis of pneumothorax, endobronchial intubation, inadvertent extubation, or a blocked endotracheal tube more difficult. Observation and palpation for chest movement and tracheal shift are useful in this regard. Passage of an endotracheal suction catheter can unblock a tube.

In addition, the airway pressure measured on the ventilator can give much useful information. If using pressure control ventilation the airway pressure will remain constant in the presence of a blocked tube, endobronchial intubation, or pneumothorax, but will fall in the presence of a displaced tube, or disconnected ventilator circuit. End tidal CO_2 monitoring is very sensitive but not very specific, but can be a helpful extra safety monitor.

If a pneumothorax develops during transport then it must be decompressed urgently. This is best done by needle thoracocentesis, as it is not practical to insert an intercostal drain during flight. However, an intercostal drain should be inserted as soon as the patient arrives at the hospital. Patients with undrained pneumothoraces should not be taken into the air until intercostal drains have been inserted, as such air spaces expand with altitude as the surrounding barometric pressure decreases. For the same reasons a nasogastric tube should be inserted to decompress the stomach. Expansion of a gastric gas bubble can act to splint the diaphragm and also decrease venous return, thereby impairing cardiovascular function.

If venous access fails in the air then the intraosseous route is the preferred technique to re-establish access to the circulation. Maintenance of core temperature is vital during transport and it is prudent to have chemically activated warming pads available in case of incubator battery failure (or expiry). The blood glucose should also be checked regularly during the flight.

- If it can fall out, it will fall out.
- If you have to ask yourself "Is central venous access needed?"—it is.
- Have you got enough oxygen?
- Is the baby warm?
- Is the blood glucose OK?

Due to the isolated nature and potential physiological effects of the aeromedical environment, staff selection is even more important than usual. Air sickness can be disabling and staff who are prone to this should not undertake air transfers if antiemetics do not control their symptoms. Staff should be specifically trained in aeromedical transfer, and this training should include a period of preceptored practice where the trainee undertakes a number of transfers accompanied by a trainer. However, there is currently no UK standard for training in aeromedical transfer for physicians or nurses, although a number of courses are available.

High altitude physiology

There are two important principles which must be remembered when transporting patients by air (see chapter 2). The first is that the total barometric pressure decreases with altitude, for instance from 760 mmHg at sea level to 565 mmHg at 2500 m (the effective altitude inside the pressurised cabin of an airliner flying at 11 000 m). This has profound effects on oxygen transport across the alveolar capillary membrane. Obviously if the patient's Fio$_2$ at sea level is, for example, 50% then the same oxygen

pressure in the alveolus can be achieved by increasing the Fio$_2$. The alveolar–arterial oxygen diffusion gradient is thereby maintained.

- In the example of the patient in 50% oxygen, alveolar oxygen pressure at sea level is 760 mmHg × 50% = 380 mmHg.
- If total atmospheric pressure at 2500 m is 565 mmHg, then 380 mmHg is equivalent to an Fio$_2$ of (380/565) × 100% = 67%.

In practice it is not necessary to perform this calculation; the Fio$_2$ can be increased until the oxygen saturation is well maintained, but the principle involved should always be remembered. The reduction in atmospheric pressure becomes more problematical when a patient is breathing 100% O$_2$ at sea level and is already hypoxic. In these patients other techniques must be used to improve oxygenation such as increasing the mean airway pressure, increasing the positive end expiratory pressure (PEEP), inverse I : E ratios (to increase mean airway pressure (MAP)) or even prone ventilation to optimise V : Q matching. It should be ensured that patients have an adequate haematocrit as anaemia may further decrease oxygen transport to life threatening levels. Patients may need transfusing prior to transport. Arguments that transfused blood is deficient in 2,3-DPG and will therefore have less efficient oxygen transport than the patient's red cells are entirely correct. It should be remembered, however, that transfused blood still carries much more oxygen than plasma, and thus it is still a useful therapeutic manoeuvre in this setting.

The other important principle is that gas filled spaces such as a pneumothorax, endotracheal tube cuff, or stomach will expand as the barometric pressure reduces with altitude. It is essential therefore that any such collections are adequately drained prior to take off. Endotracheal tube cuffs may either be filled with saline (which will not expand as much), or can have some air removed during ascent to reduce the pressure and volume. It should also be ensured that all plaster casts and constricting bandages are split down to the skin as limbs also tend to expand and can become critically ischaemic if strangulated by a cast.

One final physiological point which may become important on longer flights is the reduction in ambient humidity at altitude, which is further reduced by air conditioning. Endotracheal secretions may become inspissated, and regular endotracheal suctioning may be required. The decreased humidity also leads to greatly increased insensible fluid losses during long flights, and maintenance fluids should be adjusted to take account of this.

- Oxygen pressure falls with altitude so the Fio_2 must be increased.
- Gases and tissues expand with altitude.
- Do not take a child into the air with an undrained pneumothorax as it will expand.

Summary

Air transport can be used either to move patients long distances or to reduce transport times when moving unstable patients over shorter distances. It is usually faster to use road transport if the estimated transport time is less than two hours.

The ABC approach should be used as an aid to diagnosis, treatment, and equipment provision. This coupled with a fatalistic attitude (if it can go wrong, it will go wrong) will usually prevent complications, or ensure that they can be adequately dealt with if they arise.

The physiological problems caused by hypoxia at altitude and expansion of air spaces and body parts should be offset by drainage of pneumothoraces, insertion of a nasogastric tube, and splitting of plaster splints to allow expansion of limbs. Approximately twice as much oxygen as you think is necessary should be carried.

Safety is very important, and staff should obey the instructions of aircrew at all times. Helicopters should only be approached from the front, after permission has been given. Beware of the rotors.

Finally wrap up warm, don't forget some antiemetics and a credit card (you may get stranded), and enjoy the ride.

Part 2
Practical transport management

6 Neonatal resuscitation and stabilisation

Objective
This chapter details issues in the assessment, stabilisation and transfer of neonatal patients. Emphasis is placed on factors that distinguish the neonatal population, in particular maintenance of body temperature and transfers of babies with congenital abnormalities.

The principles of effective transport detailed throughout this manual should be as rigorously and thoughtfully applied to neonates as to any other group. This chapter is concerned with issues which may need additional attention in the transport of neonatal intensive care (NICU) patients.

Most interhospital transfers of NICU patients are of well stabilised infants who require specialist care beyond that available in the referring unit. The need for active resuscitation and substantial stabilisation will be unusual. The goal of careful pretransfer stabilisation is a baby in a safe condition for the transfer.

Who should go?

- A nurse with transport training and experience.
- A doctor at specialist registrar level or above, or an advanced neonatal nurse practitioner (ANNP), also with transport training and experience.

Assessment and stabilisation of the sick neonate

On arrival at the referring unit listen carefully to a handover, and ensure you are aware of all the necessary information.

Assess and stabilise:

- Airway
- Breathing
- Circulation
- Feeds and fluids
- Central nervous system
- Temperature.

Assessment of the respiratory system

Assess for tachypnoea, recession (intercostal/subcostal), grunting, and for apnoeas and desaturations. Assess trends in oxygen requirement and blood gases and review chest x ray films for pathology and positions of tubes and lines.

Transilluminate the chest if pneumothorax is a possibility and no chest x ray film is available. It is more difficult to detect a pneumothorax using transillumination in larger babies and confident diagnosis may be improved by taking measures to make the environment as dark as possible before transillumination.

If already intubated, assess chest movement (quantity, equality), breath sounds, and the degree of synchrony between infant and ventilator. Assess the endotracheal tube (ETT). It must be correctly positioned, secure, and patent. Do not reintubate if the ETT is secure, correctly positioned, and patent. ETTs must be secured to a high standard to avoid becoming dislodged during transfer.

Stabilisation of the respiratory system

Have a lower threshold for intubation than on the NICU, to minimise the potential for needing to intervene in transit. In an infant of more than 30 weeks' gestation if the vital signs (pulse, blood pressure, respiratory rate, temperature) and examination have been consistently stable in oxygen < 50% and if the $P\text{co}_2$ is normal, it may be acceptable to move the infant without intubation.

If the infant:

- Is unstable
- Has a rising oxygen requirement > 50%
- Is struggling to breathe (recession, grunting, head bobbing, tracheal tug)
- Has a rising $P\text{co}_2$
- Has recurrent apnoea
- Is less than 30 weeks' gestation

then intubation and respiratory support are highly likely to be required, at least for the duration of the journey.

It may be necessary to change ventilation mode for transfer, as most transport ventilators do not have facilities for high frequency oscillation or patient triggered modes. Stabilise the infant on the altered mode of ventilation before transferring to the transport system.

Use surfactant if indicated—do not delay until after transfer. Give surfactant early in the stabilisation period and manage any consequent short term instability.

Drain all pneumothoraces of babies on positive pressure ventilation before the journey, as an undrained small pneumothorax can become larger.

All ETTs should be suctioned prior to transfer to help minimise the need for intervention in transit.

Use blood gas analysis to review the results of all alterations to respiratory support. It may be necessary to site a peripheral or umbilical arterial line. Calibrate transcutaneous gas monitoring against a blood gas sample for the transfer. This is a useful tool for gauging trends and for making ventilatory adjustments in transit.

Provide adequate opiate sedation for all intubated infants. Muscle relaxation is not routinely indicated for transfer.

Aim to transfer when:

- pH 7·25–7·4 and stable or improving
- $Pa\text{CO}_2$ 4–6 kPa and stable or improving
- $Pa\text{O}_2$ 6–10 kPa and stable or improving.

- Have a low index of suspicion of the need for intubation/respiratory support.
- Stabilise the respiratory system thoroughly.

Assessment of the cardiovascular system

Assess both absolute values and trends in heart rate, colour, capillary refill time, and peripheral perfusion. These may all help diagnose impending shock.

Blood pressure may be satisfactory if the mean BP is greater than gestation in the newborn. It may be necessary to place an arterial line to assess this. The base deficit may be elevated (> 5) where there is poor perfusion. Assess the urine output, which should be more than 1 ml/kg/h, by placing a urinary catheter if necessary.

Review the haemoglobin level and arrange transfusion if the level is below 12 g/dl in sick infants.

Stabilisation of the cardiovascular system

Take a proactive approach, aiming to treat any current problems as well as ensuring that monitoring will detect problems in transit.

Place an arterial line for blood pressure monitoring if you are concerned about cardiovascular status. Avoid reliance on non-invasive blood pressure measurements in sick infants, as these are less accurate and technically challenging in transit.

Treat hypotension with volume expansion (4·5% human albumin solution or normal saline, or blood if the haemoglobin is low) 10–20 ml/kg over 30–60 minutes initially. Start inotropes if response to volume is not adequate and place a central venous line for administration.

Ensure in all circumstances you have a maternal blood sample for cross-matching after the transfer.

- Thoroughly assess cardiovascular values and trends. Place an arterial line if worried about blood pressure.
- Use volume replacement and inotropes early, as indicated. Shock and hypotension are very likely to worsen in transit.

Assessment of feeds and fluids

Check the blood glucose and recheck often when there has been instability or vascular access problems. Review serum electrolytes (U&E) and examine the abdomen for distension, tenderness or discolouration. Review whether and how recently any enteral feeds have been given.

Stabilisation of feeds and fluids

Stop enteral feeds for journeys. Place and aspirate a nasogastric tube (NGT). Ensure there is reliable IV access and administer maintenance fluids according to local policy and U&E results. Keep the blood glucose higher than 2·4 mmol/l.

Assessment of central nervous system

Review ante-, peri-, and postnatal histories for evidence of CNS injury. Observe unsedated infants for posture, tone, and activity. Where there is the possibility of CNS injury observe for subtle and/or overt signs of convulsions. Subtle signs may include sucking and chewing, cycling movements of arms and legs, and apnoea. Frank fits, tonic and/or clonic, may also be seen.

Promptly investigate seizures—check the blood glucose, U&E, calcium and magnesium. Complete a septic screen, including lumbar puncture. Collect urine as part of the septic screen—some should go for culturing as usual, but retain a sample for potential later investigations.

Stabilisation of central nervous system

Treat according to the results of investigations, to correct an underlying disorder, such as hypoglycaemia or meningitis. Definitive diagnosis and management may have to wait until after transfer. Anticonvulsants may be necessary to treat prolonged seizures (see chapter 13), but may cause respiratory depression mandating ventilation for transfer.

Current research is concerned with therapeutic hypothermia in the first hours of life for infants suffering a perinatal hypoxic/ischaemic insult, and this may be a future transport challenge.

Thermoregulation

Very immature and low birthweight babies are particularly vulnerable to cold. There is substantial evidence that transported babies are at particular risk of becoming hypothermic, and that this is associated with poor outcome. These infants represent a unique transport challenge, and every effort must be made to promote normothermia. The following advice refers in particular to infants of weights less than < 1·5 kg, but the principles should be generally applied to neonatal transfers.

Before setting off to retrieve a low birthweight baby

Obtain information about the current temperature of the baby, and offer advice to the referring team, if required. Prewarm the transport incubator to 39–40°C. It may be necessary to run the transport incubator at its top setting as heat is lost much more rapidly to the environment on a transfer than in a well heated NICU.

Some transport incubators may be humidified using a simple wet sponge device—start this process now.

During stabilisation on the referring unit

Ensure the transport incubator is plugged in and warming. Monitor the infant's temperature continuously with a sensor placed in a core position such as under the infant or fixed with a spot plaster in the axilla.

Nurse the infant in a warm, humidified incubator. Bubblewrap may help reduce evaporative heat loss. Actively warm and humidify ventilator gases. Rewarming may be helped by use of a chemically activated gel mattress (Advanced Health Technologies, Herts, UK) to provide an additional source of heat when placed under the infant.

Refractory hypothermia may respond to placing the whole baby in a headbox with warmed gas flow via a humidifier, as for headbox oxygen.

Do not transfer to the transport incubator until the temperature is normal, or at least improving. The need for rewarming and/or maintaining temperature should be factored into the timing of stabilisation procedures. It may be necessary to apply some of the rewarming procedures above for some time before placing tubes or lines that are needed for the transfer.

Transfer to the transport incubator

Time spent in transfer from the hospital isolette to the transport incubator will exacerbate heat loss due to time spent in contact with cooler air. This transfer should be completed in a maximum of 15 seconds, timed from opening the doors of the static incubator to closing the doors of the transport incubator.

The infant may be conveyed between incubators on an activated chemical warming mattress. Complete all subsequent procedures through portholes.

Humidify ventilator gases for transfer. A simple heat and moisture exchanger is probably as effective as active humidification for transfer.

Before leaving for return journey

Minimise the need for any intervention requiring opening portholes during the journey by ensuring all monitoring is properly attached and working, and all tubes and lines are patent before departing.

Return journey

Warm the ambulance cabin. Attempt to complete the journey without opening the incubator portholes. Monitor temperature continuously and adjust the incubator accordingly.

In the event of deterioration of the clinical condition requiring active intervention, balance the likelihood of profound hypothermia consequent on performing a definitive procedure against the possibility of performing a limited procedure in the vehicle and diverting to a nearby hospital, where treatment may be completed and temperature protected.

> • Special attention must be paid to thermo-regulation on transfer of preterm and low birthweight babies, as this affects outcome.
> • Meticulous attention to detail is necessary to keep small babies warm before and during transfer.
> • Protecting thermal status should be factored into all clinical decisions.

Care of the family

The transport team should consider care of the infant's family to be a central part of their work. After initial introductions, it is best if the team members can each set aside some time with the family during the stabilising period. Establish what the family already understand about their baby's illness and the need for transfer, and build on this established knowledge to ensure they are aware of the key current problems, treatments, and transport issues. Written and other information for the family is helpful at this stage, and many transport teams carry pre-prepared materials tailored to the local arrangements.

Discuss the family's travel arrangements and make sure you have all the necessary phone numbers to contact them if necessary.

Acute deterioration and resuscitation of the newborn

The need for cardiopulmonary resuscitation of neonates by transport teams should be rare. In the situation where two or more personnel are dedicated to the care of one infant most problems may be managed before they become a crisis.

Endeavour to keep infants warm throughout resuscitation. As far as possible perform procedures through the incubator portholes. Use bubblewrap and heated chemical gel mattresses early in the process.

Infants will usually present with a combination of desaturation and/or bradycardia.

Airway and breathing

In unintubated infants check for breathing. Support respirations with bag-valve-mask ventilation, checking that chest movement is achieved. If the chest does not move (re-evaluate this after each step):

• Ensure the head is in the neutral position
• Ensure there is a good seal of the mask over the infant's mouth and nose
• Consider using a Guedel airway or jaw thrust
• Intubate.

In intubated infants check for chest movement. If none:

• Check the ventilator is delivering breaths and has not become disconnected
• Suction down the ETT
• Reintubate if concerned the ETT is blocked or dislodged
• Assess for pneumothorax—see below.

If the chest is moving:

• Assess the quality of chest movement—if reduced, does the baby need higher pressures or a faster rate? If the baby is fighting the ventilator increase the dose of sedation and consider muscle relaxation. Check the IV line delivering sedation has not dislodged
• Assess for pneumothorax with transillumination and chest radiograph. Needle thoracocentesis and/or chest drain placement will be necessary if pneumothorax is present.

Circulation

In the situation where, despite adequate ventilation and good chest movement, the heart rate is less than around 60 beats/min, start chest compressions.

The most effective method is encircling the chest with both hands and using the thumbs to compress the lower third of the sternum (Fig. 6.1). The thumbs should be just below an imaginary line joining the nipples. Aim to compress the lower third of the sternum by about one third the depth of the chest. Current neonatal resuscitation guidelines suggest aiming to achieve 90 compressions and 30 breaths per minute, in a ratio of three compressions to each breath.

Chest compressions may be sufficient to move oxygenated blood the short distance from the pulmonary bed to the coronary arteries, and so restore a normal heart rate. If not, consider using resuscitation drugs.

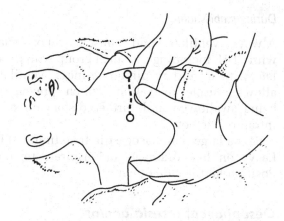

Figure 6.1 Chest compressions. (From Resuscitation Council, UK. *Newborn Life Support Provider Course Manual.* London: Resuscitation Council, 2001, with permission. Illustration by Steven Brindley.)

The evidence for when and how to use resuscitation drugs in the newborn is poor. There is broad agreement of the four drugs that may be used, but not the order in which to use them. Familiarise yourself with local policy and follow that.

Sodium bicarbonate 4·2%

Dose: 1–2 mmol/kg (2–4 ml/kg)
Route: UVC or other venous line.

- To improve the intracardiac biochemical milieu to allow the heart to work normally. Follow the dose with a small 0·9% saline flush and continue compressions for a brief period before reassessing heart rate.

Epinephrine (adrenaline) 1 : 10 000

Dose: 10 micrograms/kg (0·1 ml/kg 1 : 10 000)
Route: UVC, other venous line or via tracheal tube.

- As adrenaline may not be effective when the pH is low, it may be worth giving a further dose of 0·3 ml/kg of 1 : 10 000 solution after a dose of bicarbonate if there was no response to an earlier dose.
- Unlike the other resuscitation drugs, epinephrine may be safely given down the tracheal tube. The current recommendation is to give the same dose as the IV route.

Dextrose 10%

Dose: 2·5 ml/kg
Route: UVC or other venous line.

- Supplies a bolus of fuel to the heart when glycogen stores may have diminished.

Volume (normal saline/4·5% human albumin solution/blood)

Dose: 10 ml/kg initially
Route: UVC or other venous line.

- Rarely bradycardia will respond to volume. Give 10 ml/kg and assess response.
- Do not give more than 10–20 ml/kg volume expansion unless there is evidence of loss of fluid from the circulation, for example from a disconnected UVC/UAC, fluid loss into the abdomen from bowel perforation or large intraventricular haemorrhage.

Resuscitation in transit

First, stop the ambulance. Take immediate steps to warm the vehicle cabin (close windows, turn the vehicle heater on full) to improve the baby's thermal environment if procedures such as intubation are necessary.

At each stage it will be necessary to balance the need for a definitive procedure, such as chest drain placement, against the risk of performing the procedure in a cold environment with limited help. Consider performing a limited procedure, such as needle thoracocentesis, and diverting to the nearest hospital in order to do the definitive procedure in a warm and controlled environment.

Use the mobile phone if necessary to seek senior advice, particularly if resuscitation attempts are proving unsuccessful. In the event of unsuccessful resuscitation it may be best to take the baby to whichever hospital the parents are at.

Congenital abnormalities and transfers for neonatal surgery

This section outlines specific issues, beyond normal transport practice, that need consideration for these groups of infants.

Gastroschisis/exomphalos

Before departing to retrieve an infant with gastroschisis

Ensure you have an appropriate plastic bag to nurse the baby in, for example Vi-Drape Intestinal Bag (Becton Dickinson, Meylon, France), as well as adequate supplies of volume replacement fluids (for example, human albumin solution 4·5%). Infants with gastroschisis may need 20–60 ml/kg in the first six hours.

During stabilisation

Inspect the defect. Even if it has been carefully, thoroughly and recently covered with a dressing, this should be removed and not replaced. Nurse in a clear plastic bag, secured under the arms. Signs of ischaemia (black, poorly perfused bowel) should be discussed urgently by telephone with the surgeon at the receiving unit. Anecdotally, it is said to be very occasionally necessary to enlarge the abdominal wall defect to restore perfusion to the bowel.

Maintain circulating volume now and during the journey by estimating fluid losses from the defect and replacing. Volume status may be assessed by:

- Trends in blood pressure and capillary refill
- Aspirating and measuring exudate from the plastic bag. This needs aspirating regularly to help keep baby dry
- Worsening toe/core temperature gap trend.

Position baby and defect carefully to prevent stretching or twisting of the mesentery. Large defects may need supporting.

Infants with a covered exomphalos are much more straightforward to transfer.

Congenital diaphragmatic hernia

Infants with congenital diaphragmatic hernia (CDH) are often extremely unwell, and require prompt, effective and thorough general intensive care to stabilise for transfer.

Before departing to retrieve an infant with CDH

Consider taking inhaled nitric oxide on the transfer. Be prepared for a complex transfer, with potentially many infusions.

During stabilisation

Always ventilate and muscle relax infants with CDH, including the small group who present late with a mild respiratory illness. Ventilation allows muscle relaxation, which prevents air being swallowed and further distension of the intrathoracic bowel.

Pass a large bore nasogastric tube (min. 10 FG). Leave on free drainage and aspirate regularly. Position hernia side down.

Oesophageal atresia and/or tracheo-oesophageal fistula

Infants with tracheo-oesophageal fistula (TOF) will usually be straightforward to transfer. If there is an oesophageal atresia, a replogle tube (Sherwood Medical, Tullamore, Rep. Ireland) should be placed in the oesophageal pouch. These double lumen tubes have a large lumen for aspirating pouch contents and a smaller second lumen for instilling small amounts of normal saline regularly to loosen secretions. They are sufficiently rigid not to curl up in the pouch. Position the infant slightly head up, to encourage secretions to pool in the pouch, from where they may be aspirated.

Ventilation for transfer should be avoided in this group. Babies with oesophageal atresia (OA) and a distal fistula are a unique ventilation problem. Massive irreducible abdominal distension is likely to follow from positive pressure ventilation and this may lead to a vicious cycle of increasing abdominal distension, thoracic compression, and worsening respiratory state. If ventilation has already been started, or is unavoidable, transfer should proceed very promptly and the receiving surgical and anaesthetic teams notified.

Bowel obstruction and other gastrointestinal pathology

Bowel obstruction in the newborn requires transfer for paediatric surgical assessment and management. In many cases definitive diagnosis is not possible until after transfer and so the work of the transport team is to carefully assess the baby and offer the support necessary to allow for a safe journey. Potential diagnoses include bowel atresia, meconium ileus, malrotation/volvulus, Hirschsprung's disease, and necrotising enterocolitis (NEC). Some may be complicated by perforation of the bowel.

Considerations for transfer

Is there a need for urgent transfer? Babies with bowel perforation and/or malrotation need prompt surgical assessment. The time spent on very thorough stabilisation for transfer should be balanced against the possibility of life saving surgery.

Always place a large bore NGT, leave it on free drainage, and aspirate regularly. If fluid management has been adequate in the preceding period, then replacement fluids are rarely required in transit. Replacement of NG losses may be necessary if these have not been replaced prior to arrival of the transport team. Normal saline will usually be adequate replacement fluid for transfer.

Assess for serum electrolyte disturbances but, unless transfer will take several hours, do not delay transfer of a critically ill baby in order to calculate electrolyte deficits and mix custom fluid bags.

For babies with NEC, and other painful conditions, consider administration of opiate analgesia. This may also necessitate ventilation, but this is better and safer practice than transferring an infant who keeps going apnoeic through pain.

Consent

Ensure that arrangements are made for proper consent for surgery to be obtained by the surgeon from an eligible person. As valid informed consent may only be obtained by a senior member of the surgical team, it is not appropriate for the transport team to seek consent. Instead, the transport team should seek to ensure that consent is facilitated. Consider:

- When the infant will go to surgery—infants with perforated bowel, for example, may need an urgent procedure soon after transfer, whereas many infants with diaphragmatic hernia are stabilised for several days
- When a person who is able to give valid consent will be able to come to the surgical centre.

Balance these two factors. The best solution is for a parent to meet the surgeon before the surgery.

In the event that emergency surgery will be needed on completion of transfer and it is not possible for a consent giver to travel at this time, it may be necessary for the transport team to facilitate and witness a telephone conversation between the surgeon and the consent giver.

Transfer from the labour ward and other intrahospital transfers

In many hospitals there is a substantial distance between labour ward and the NICU, necessitating a carefully planned approach to this transfer. In addition, infants who need surgery and investigations may have to leave the NICU while critically ill. The latter group should be prepared for transfer exactly as for an interhospital transfer.

The approach to transfers from labour ward to the NICU is determined by the distance involved and by the presence of significant obstacles, such as lifts. If the transfer time is routinely more than a minute or two, a transport incubator should be used in preference to the Resuscitaire.

Whatever the distance involved, the principles described below should be observed.

Keep the baby warm. Where a transport incubator is to be used, it should be kept warm at all times. As well as conventional warming methods, such as use of the Resuscitaire, chemical gel mattresses and woolly hats, recent data suggest that putting newborn infants in a plastic bag up to the neck immediately at birth is effective in retaining heat, presumably by reducing evaporative heat loss. The bag is left in place until the infant is settled on the NICU.

Attend thoroughly to airway, breathing, and circulation, and ensure you have control of these for the transfer. If intubation has been necessary, secure the tube. Administer surfactant if indicated. Ensure the baby's chest is moving. If using the transport incubator, attach the infant to the ventilator so that the incubator portholes can be kept closed.

Neonatal procedures

Umbilical vessel catheterisation

The umbilical vessels provide ready access to the central venous and arterial circulations. Elective umbilical catheterisation should be approached as a sterile procedure.

Equipment

- Sterile procedure pack (including artery forceps and vessel probes), gown, gloves
- Cord ligature

- Scalpel and large blade
- Syringes and saline flushes
- Suitable catheters for vessels:

  - Umbilical vein—size 5–10FG single or double lumen
  - Umbilical artery—size 3·5–5FG single lumen; some have oxygen measuring electrodes at the tip
  - Three-way taps for catheters, to allow subsequent sampling
  - Blood pressure monitoring circuit for arterial lines.

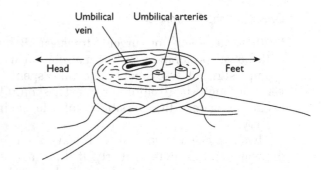

Figure 6.2 Orientation and appearance of umbilical vessels when the umbilical cord is cut close to the level of the skin. The arteries are small, thick walled, and may stand proud of the cut surface. The vein is large and thin walled. (From Resuscitation Council, UK. *Newborn Life Support Provider Course Manual.* London: Resuscitation Council, 2001, with permission. Illustration by Steven Brindley.)

Procedure

- Using aseptic procedure, clean the cord and periumbilical skin and drape the area.
- Attach three-way taps to catheters and prime catheter(s) with normal saline.
- Tie an umbilical cord ligature loosely around the base of the cord. This may be pulled tight to control bleeding.
- Cut the umbilical cord 1–2 cm above the skin. Cut cleanly, avoiding a sawing motion.
- Identify the three vessels (Fig. 6.2).
- For umbilical vein:

  - Use an artery forceps to grip one wall of the vein. The vein may need to be gently dilated with a probe, but most often will not.
  - Gently insert the catheter. Some resistance may be felt at the umbilical ring—gentle pressure may be applied to pass the catheter beyond this point.
  - Advance the catheter—it should not be passed further than the distance from the cord base to the internipple line.
  - Draw back on the syringe—if blood is readily aspirated the catheter is in a large vessel and is probably in an adequate position for transport. If blood is not aspirated, try withdrawing or advancing the catheter slightly.

- For umbilical artery:

  - Stabilise the cord stump by placing two artery forceps tangentially to the cord, one on each side.
  - Carefully dilate the lumen of one of the arteries to a depth of 5 mm, using a fine pair of forceps to tease open the vessel, or a blunt dilator.

- Insert the catheter tip into the dilated vessel and advance the catheter. Blood should be readily obtained on aspiration. The catheter tip needs to rest at a position that avoids the origins of the renal artery, coeliac axis, or inferior mesenteric artery. Obtain an *x* ray picture to ensure the tip of the catheter is either between T8 and T10 or L3 and L4.
- Observe the infant for the development of signs of distal hypoperfusion—blue or white legs, or blue toes. If these occur the catheter should be promptly removed. Try again, either in the other artery or with a smaller catheter.

The umbilical vein may be cannulated on transfer when central venous access is required, either for infusion of vasoactive drugs such as inotropes, or where other venous access proves difficult, such as in very poorly perfused infants. Double lumen catheters increase the utility of the vessel, providing two separate vascular access routes. Consider the umbilical vein in babies up to 10–14 days of age where there is any dried up umbilical cord stump remaining adherent. Follow the procedure above, but expose the vessel in the following manner.

- Grip the umbilical cord stump with toothed forceps and apply gentle traction.
- Use the blade to cut off the dried up cord stump as close to the base as possible without cutting skin.
- The vein should be exposed in the superior position and may be cannulated as above.

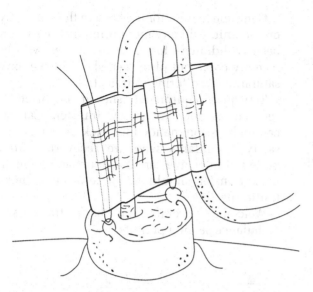

Figure 6.3 Securing umbilical lines. Tie two stitches into the substance of the umbilical cord and cut the silk about 4 cm long. Line these ends up alongside the catheter and then turn the catheter back on itself and tape all together so that silk and catheter are encased in the tape. Use very sticky pink tape ("Sleek") and avoid tape on skin. (From Resuscitation Council, UK. *Newborn Life Support Provider Course Manual.* London: Resuscitation Council, 2001, with permission. Illustration by Steven Brindley.)

- Be prepared to control bleeding from the stump either with direct pressure or, if the bleeding is from the vein, by applying pressure to the abdomen 1–2 cm directly superior to the cord. A haemostatic dressing (for example, Surgicel) is also occasionally required.

For transfer ensure that the catheter is very secure (Fig. 6.3); a displaced UVC may lead to rapid substantial blood loss. Once you have secured the catheter, verify its security by gently pulling on it—it should not move. Chest and abdominal radiographs are needed to check the position of tips of lines and verify that the desired vessels were cannulated.

Peripheral arterial cannulation is probably preferable to placing a UAC for transfer, simply as it's a quicker procedure that does not require an *x* ray film afterwards. However, where peripheral arterial cannulation has not been possible and accurate blood pressure measurement is required, then placing a UAC may be necessary. The umbilical arteries are not usually accessible beyond the first 2–3 days of life.

> Do not delay necessary tasks until after the transfer—if you are wondering whether it needs doing, it probably does.

Back transfer

Neonatal intensive care is distinctive in the provision of care right through to hospital discharge. Back transfer to a hospital that is local for the infant's family should happen as soon as it is safe. The principles of safe back transfer are the same as for any other transfer, as detailed elsewhere in this chapter. Below are some brief additional considerations.

Planning back transfer

Back transfer should normally be a planned activity. Start this planning from the time of admission by discussing it with the infant's family. Ensure they understand that their baby will be returned to a local unit at some point, and explore any issues that arise from this. All staff should avoid any discussion which elevates the status of tertiary units relative to local units in their ability to provide care—it is all too easy to make parents wrongly believe that their local unit is incapable of caring for their baby. Keep in contact with the local unit to ensure they are aware that there is a baby who will be returning to them at some point.

Local agreements and circumstances determine whether back transfer is performed by the tertiary or local hospital. In either case, it is crucial that the two units cooperate on a collaborative approach to return transfers.

Concrete plans for back transfer should be actively constructed from as soon as the period of acute illness appears to be ending. The tertiary centre should contact the local unit to alert them to the impending transfer, and to discuss timing.

For babies who have needed ventilation avoid plans that involve extubation followed by imminent back transfer, especially in premature infants. It is better to electively leave the infant intubated for transfer, with a plan for weaning and extubation promptly at the local centre, than to extubate and transfer soon after. Recently extubated infants may find the handling and stress associated with back transfer excessive, and need reventilating. The alternative is to extubate and leave the baby for a day or two before transferring.

Back transfer should include the transfer of all the information necessary for the local unit to continue the care of the baby. Local agreements determine what this comprises, in terms of letters, copies of notes, *x* ray films and so on, and these should be prepared well ahead of time.

Who should go?

Back transfers without exception need a nurse who is experienced in transport. This is to ensure that all the safety-in-transit issues are properly attended to, the transport equipment is used effectively, and clinical deteriorations are both spotted early and attended to safely.

Some back transfers, including those of ventilated infants and those in high concentrations of oxygen, require a doctor or ANNP in addition to the nurse.

Practical considerations

Stop continuous NGT feeds one hour before transfer and aspirate the tube to empty the stomach. For all but the shortest transfers infants on continuous feeds will need an IV glucose solution.

Babies on intermittent feeds may not need IV fluids, depending substantially on how long the journey is and what the feeding frequency is. For example, an infant being fed four hourly who is stable and going on a 30 minute transfer will probably not need IV fluids.

Check the blood glucose prior to departure and ensure all tubes and lines are secure and patent.

Continue to monitor the baby in the same way as on the unit. Add any monitoring that has recently been withdrawn—for example, babies who have recently come out of oxygen should have oxygen saturation monitoring in transit.

Transport equipment should be used and secured as for emergency transfer. Car seats cannot be recommended for back transfer, as their safety for infants who are recovering from a period of intensive care has not been established. Back transfer should be undertaken at normal traffic speeds.

Welcome parent(s) on back transfers, as ambulance seating permits.

Summary
In common with other groups, neonatal patients should be thoroughly stabilised for transfer.
Additional attention to maintaining body temperature is required.
There are distinctive issues in transferring infants with prematurity, congenital abnormalities or for neonatal surgery, with which the transport team must be familiar.

7 Paediatric resuscitation and stabilisation

Objectives
To recognise and take appropriate actions in the event of impending or actual cardiorespiratory arrest.
To know the observations and interventions that need to be considered to stabilise the patient before departure.
To have an understanding of the procedures described, leading to an ability to undertake them with further practice.

In most retrievals, the patient will have been resuscitated and stabilised by the referring team. The retrieval centre has an important role in optimising this phase by giving advice and identifying specific interventions that can be initiated by the referring hospital before the retrieval personnel arrive, such as intubating the child, getting vascular access, or starting inotropes. The importance of maintaining clear lines of communication between the referring team and the retrieval personnel at the time of the initial referral and *during the time spent travelling to the patient* has already been mentioned and deserves emphasis.

Occasionally, however, the child will not be stable on the retrieval team's arrival, perhaps because specific advice was not given, because the referring personnel were unable to initiate the suggested management plan, or because the child has deteriorated further. On other occasions, the child will deteriorate during transport, despite your best efforts. For this reason, retrieval personnel must have advanced life support skills and must be highly competent in paediatric resuscitation. This chapter reviews resuscitation guidelines, outlines the critical actions that must be taken before leaving the referring hospital, and finally describes some of the procedures that may be undertaken.

Much of the information needed is in other chapters of this manual (especially chapters 8 and 9), to which the reader is referred where appropriate.

Recognition and assessment of the sick child

First undertake a rapid assessment of the child, to determine whether any immediate intervention is needed (Box 7.1). Your detailed assessment should then follow a systematic approach, as outlined in the various paediatric life support manuals available.

The two facts underlying your approach to resuscitation are:

- Most cardiac arrests in children are due to hypoxia
- The outcome is generally poor once the child arrests.

Therefore you should identify the signs that the child is at risk of cardiorespiratory collapse before it happens and intervene appropriately. It is axiomatic that you need to know the normal range of physiological parameters at different ages.

Assessment of the respiratory system

Noisy breathing

This is normally due to obstruction to the flow of air, either by secretions at the back of the throat, upper airway obstruction, such as croup, or lower airway obstruction, as in acute asthma. In general, inspiratory noise (stridor) is due to upper airway obstruction. The loudness of the noise is *not* an indicator of severity, which is best assessed by the degree of recession, and the presence of pulsus paradoxus. Cyanosis due to upper airway obstruction indicates severe obstruction, and impending respiratory collapse. A scheme for the assessment and treatment of the child with croup is given in Table 7.1.

Other causes of upper airway obstruction, such as epiglottitis and foreign body, should be considered. If epiglottitis is a possibility, the airway should be secured in the referring hospital

Box 7.1   Rapid cardiopulmonary assessment

A.   AIRWAY PATENCY

B.   BREATHING

Rate:

	Newborn	1 year	18 years
	< 40	24	16

(> 60 "always" abnormal)

Air entry: Chest rise, breath sounds, stridor, wheezing
Mechanics: Retractions, grunting

C.   CIRCULATION

Heart rate:

Newborn–3 months	3 months–2 years	2–10 years	> 10 years
140	130	80	75

Abnormal: < 5 years: > 180, < 60
> 5 years: > 160

Peripheral/central pulses: Present/absent, volume

Skin perfusion: Capillary refill < 3 seconds
Temperature, colour, mottling

CNS perfusion: Recognises parents, reaction to pain,
muscle tone, pupil size

Blood pressure:

	Newborn	1 year	> 1 year
Systolic	> 60	> 70	> 70 + (age × 2)

Note: Blood pressure only distinguishes compensated from uncompensated shock
ASSESS—ACT—REASSESS—REACT

Table 7.1   Assessment of croup

	Category		
	1	*2*	*3*
Stridor	Inspiratory	Biphasic	Silent
Sternal recession	Absent	Present	Severe
Pulsus paradoxus	Absent	Absent	Present

Children in category 3 should have their airway secured prior to transport.
Children in category 2 may be given nebulised epinephrine (adrenaline) and their response
assessed. It may still be safer to secure their airway prior to transfer.

in a controlled environment, with the help of an experienced anaesthetist and the availability of an ENT surgeon to secure a surgical airway if necessary.

Expiratory noise generally suggests lower respiratory obstruction, such as bronchospasm in asthma.

Grunting is also produced in exhalation, but is the noise made by breathing out against a partially closed glottis. This manoeuvre is used, typically by infants, to generate some end expiratory pressure, and thus keep the lungs open at the end of expiration.

Beware the silent child with respiratory distress. They may just be too exhausted to make any noise.

Rate and pattern of breathing

An increased rate of breathing at rest may be due to fever, fright, lung or airway disease, or metabolic acidosis. Accessory muscles may be

Table 7.2 Modified Glasgow Coma Scale

Response	Score
Eye opening	
Spontaneous	4
On command/reacts to speech	3
On pain/reacts to pain	2
No eye opening	1
Best motor response	
Spontaneous or on command	6
Localises pain	5
Flexion with pain	4
Decorticate posturing	3
Decerebrate posturing	2
No motor response	1
Best verbal response	
Smiles, orientated, follows objects or converses appropriately	5
Disorientated, consolable crying or converses inappropriately	4
Inappropriate words, cries only to pain	3
Incomprehensible, inconsolable, moans to pain	2
No verbal response to pain	1
Total	3–15

used to help expand the chest when the work of breathing is increased. Recession is also due to an increased work of breathing, and is prominent in infants, who have a more compliant chest wall. In the extreme, this may manifest as 'see-saw' respirations, where the diaphragm moves down during inspiration, pushing the abdominal wall out, but rather than expanding, the compliant chest moves in. On expiration, the reverse happens, there is no air movement, and breathing is ineffective.

Effectiveness of breathing

Chest expansion, listening for breath sounds, and oxygen saturation all give indications of the effectiveness of breathing.

Assessment of the cardiovascular system

Heart rate increases early in shock, to compensate for a falling stroke volume, and in hyperdynamic states, because infants have relatively non-compliant ventricles and are therefore less able to increase stroke volume to improve cardiac output. The peripheral pulse becomes weak and thready, and may be absent. Skin perfusion deteriorates, and a useful sign of impending shock is cold peripheries. Running the hand up the lower leg

will enable you to define a demarcation between warm and cold skin, and the level of demarcation may be used to monitor response to interventions. Capillary refill time is also used, but is more subjective.

Blood pressure is a poor sign of circulatory failure, as it is maintained until collapse is imminent. A low diastolic pressure may indicate relative hypovolaemia. It is important that the correct cuff size is used to measure blood pressure by the non-invasive method.

Finally, assess the effect of circulatory failure on end organs. Poor skin perfusion has already been mentioned. Agitation, aggression and then drowsiness may be due to poor cerebral perfusion, and poor urine output suggests inadequate renal perfusion.

Assessment of the nervous system

A deteriorating or reduced conscious level is most commonly due to reduced cerebral oxygen delivery, secondary to hypoxia or shock. Therefore optimise the airway, breathing and circulation first. Conscious level may be difficult to assess formally, especially in infants, but the AVPU system provides a simple and reproducible method of doing so (Box 7.2).

Box 7.2

A	**A**lert
V	Responds to **V**oice
P	Responds to **P**ain
U	**U**nresponsive

The traditional Glasgow Coma Scale (GCS) is modified to accommodate young children (Table 7.2). Such assessments should be repeated frequently, as conscious level may change rapidly, and are a good guide to the effectiveness of resuscitation. In general, children with a GCS less than 8 are unable to protect their airway. If simple resuscitative measures do not improve their conscious level, the airway should be secured by means of endotracheal intubation.

Raised intracranial pressure (ICP) is suggested by the following signs, *in the appropriate clinical setting*.

- Pupillary reactions—unilateral or bilateral dilatation suggests raised ICP.
- Posturing (Fig. 7.1)—a painful stimulus may be needed to elicit abnormal posturing. In

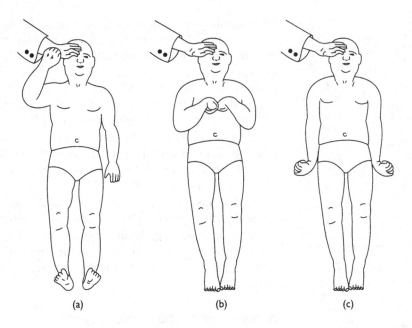

Figure 7.1 (a) Normal flexor response to pain in an unconscious patient. (b) Abnormal flexion: decorticate posturing seen in upper brainstem injury. (c) Abnormal extension: decerebrate posturing seen in lower midbrain/upper pons injury. (From Glasgow JFT, Graham HK. *Management of Injuries in Children*. London: BMJ Books, 1997.)

Table 7.3 CNS lesions by site and typical clinical observations

CNS level of lesion	Pupil reactions	Oculocephalic reflexes	Breathing pattern	Posture
Thalamus	Small, reactive	Variable	Cheyne–Stokes	Normal (A)
Midbrain	Mid position, fixed	Absent	Hyperventilation	Decorticate (B), increased tone
Pons	Pinpoint, fixed	Absent	Rhythmic pauses	Decerebrate (C) or flaccid
Medulla	Small, reactive	Present	Irregular	Flaccid

decorticate posturing the arms flex and the legs extend. In decerebrate posturing, both arms and legs extend.

• Reflexes (Table 7.3)—the oculocephalic reflexes involve flexing and rotating the head, and should not be tested in patients who may have neck trauma. The eyes should move away from the head movement when the head is rotated to the side. No movement, or random movement, is abnormal. Similarly, when the head is flexed, the eyes should deviate upwards. Loss of conjugate upward gaze is suggestive of raised ICP.

Systemic hypertension with sinus bradycardia in the obtunded patient is suggestive of cerebral herniation, and is a late and ominous sign. If the airway has not been secured, do so, ventilate to a normal CO_2 and give mannitol (0·5–1 g/kg IV). In some situations dexamethasone may be useful.

Learning points
A rapid cardiopulmonary assessment of the child should be made, following the traditional ABC approach.
Most cardiorespiratory arrests in children are due to hypoxia, and early intervention can prevent many of these.
Knowledge of the normal physiological parameters at different ages is essential to identify the abnormal.

Critical interventions

The rapid assessment or the more detailed systematic survey may reveal immediate interventions that are needed to prevent further deterioration. These should be initiated, their effects reassessed, and the full assessment completed. It is easy to get side-tracked in solving one particular problem, and then to miss others. This will be avoided by the use of the systems approach suggested below. Certain critical interventions may need to be undertaken immediately.

Establish an adequate airway

The child who is unable to protect his or her airway should be intubated and mechanically ventilated.

Support breathing

The child who is hypoventilating, or is at risk of hypoventilating, or is requiring more than 60% oxygen by face mask for transfer, should generally be intubated and mechanically ventilated.

Support the circulation

A child with hypotension or in compensated shock should have intravenous access established and be supported with the use of plasma expanders and possibly inotropes.

Treat raised intracranial pressure

If there are signs of raised ICP, secure the airway, ventilate to a normal CO_2, give mannitol (0·5–1 g/kg IV) and consider dexamethasone.

Don't ever forget glucose

Check the blood sugar, especially in the small infant with low glucose stores.

Resuscitation algorithms

The algorithms shown in Figures 7.2–7.5 are based on published guidelines. Staff responsible for the transfer of critically ill children should have training and expertise in paediatric resuscitation, and should ideally be certified paediatric life support providers.

Asystole/bradycardia (Figs 7.2, 7.3)

Hypoxia, hypotension, and acidosis are the common causes of bradycardia in children, which, unless intervention takes place, proceeds to asystole. Clearly the overall condition of the patient must be taken into account (super fit

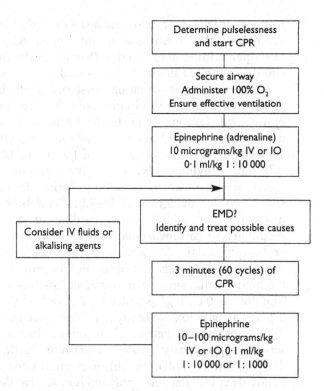

Figure 7.2 Asystole algorithm. (Adapted from Advanced Life Support Group. *Advanced Paediatric Life Support*, 3rd edn. London: BMJ Books, 2001.)

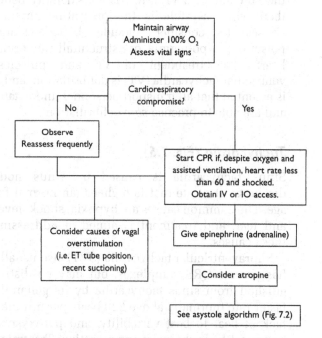

Figure 7.3 Bradycardia algorithm. (Adapted from Advanced Life Support Group. *Advanced Paediatric Life Support*, 3rd edn. London: BMJ Books, 2001.)

teenage athletes may have low heart rates that are normal for them), but a heart rate less than 60 beats per minute associated with poor perfusion should be treated in any infant or child.

As in any arrest situation, first optimise the airway, breathing, and circulation. After oxygen, epinephrine (adrenaline) is the first drug, given at a dose of 0·1 ml/kg of the 1 : 10 000 solution, with subsequent doses of 0·1 ml/kg of the 1 : 10 000 solution. Previous advice to give subsequent doses of 0·1 ml/kg of 1 : 1000 solution is not supported by evidence of benefit. The higher dose may be useful where cardiac arrest is secondary to cardiovascular collapse (i.e. sepsis or anaphylaxis). Atropine may be useful in situations where vagal stimulation has provoked the bradycardia, such as endotracheal suctioning. The dose is 0·02 mg/kg, but do not give less than 0·1 mg, as paradoxical bradycardia may occur.

The commonest causes of pulseless electrical activity (previously called electromechanical dissociation or EMD) in children are hypoxia, hypovolaemia, tension pneumothorax, cardiac tamponade, electrolyte disorders, and hypothermia. They should be actively sought and treated.

Ventricular fibrillation (Fig. 7.4)

In contrast to adults, ventricular fibrillation (VF) is an uncommon arrhythmia in children, although the outcome of a VF arrest is considerably better than when asystole is the presenting rhythm. Causes to consider include hyperkalaemia, poisoning, hypothermia, or a structurally abnormal heart. The treatment of VF and pulseless ventricular tachycardia (VT) is defibrillation, and it is essential that all transport personnel understand and are able to practise *safe* defibrillation.

Tachycardia (Fig. 7.5)

Sinus tachycardia is caused by sinus node discharge at a rate that is higher than normal for age. The common causes are hypoxia, shock, fever and fear, and treatment is aimed at addressing these causes.

Supraventricular tachycardia (SVT) also usually has narrow QRS complexes, but may be distinguished from sinus tachycardia by its generally faster rate (normally above 220 beats per minute), lack of beat to beat variability, and paroxysmal nature with abrupt onset and cessation. Treatment depends upon the condition of the child. If shock

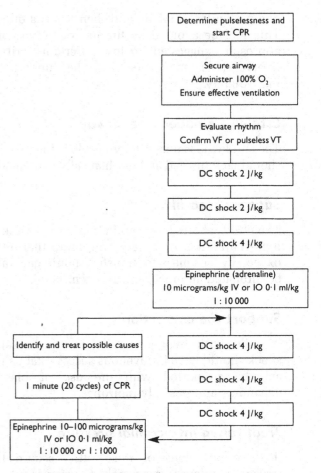

Figure 7.4 VF/pulseless VT algorithm. (Adapted from Advanced Life Support Group. *Advanced Paediatric Life Support*, 3rd edn. London: BMJ Books, 2001.)

is present, synchronised DC cardioversion should be undertaken. The initial energy level is 0·5 J/kg, increasing to 1 J/kg, and 2 J/kg on the second and third attempts if necessary.

Adenosine is the initial drug of choice in the treatment of SVT. It acts by blocking conduction at the AV node and has a very short half life and duration of effect of less than two minutes. For this reason it should be given rapidly and followed by a rapid saline bolus. The initial dose is 50 micrograms/kg, doubled if this does not work (100 micrograms/kg), and doubled again for the third dose if needed (200 micrograms/kg).

Wide complex tachycardia is most likely due to a ventricular arrhythmia, as SVT is narrow complex in 90% of cases. Again, if shock is present, synchronised DC cardioversion should be undertaken. The initial energy level is 0·5 J/kg, increasing to 1 J/kg and 2 J/kg on the second and third attempts if necessary. Amiodarone is the drug treatment of choice in VT, but treatment

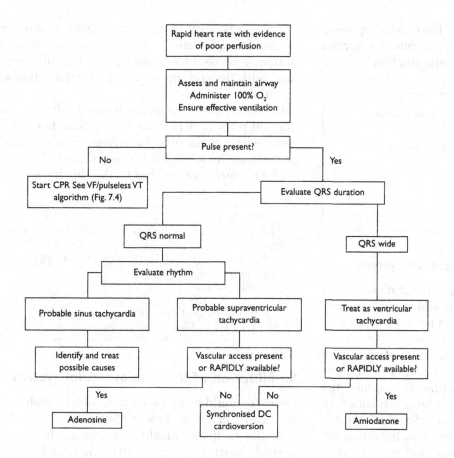

Figure 7.5 Tachycardia algorithm. (Adapted from Advanced Life Support Group. *Advanced Paediatric Life Support*, 3rd edn. London: BMJ Books, 2001.)

should normally be instigated after consultation with a paediatric cardiologist. The dose is 5 mg/kg over 30–60 minutes IV. It is important not to delay therapy for longer than necessary in VT, as this may degenerate to pulseless VT or VF. Lidocaine (lignocaine) has been used in the past. It raises the threshold for fibrillation and reduces the occurrence of postcardioversion ventricular arrhythmia. It may be given in a dose of 1 mg/kg IV, with a subsequent infusion of 20–50 micrograms/kg/min if successful. Cardioversion should not be delayed while waiting for drugs if shock is present.

Ideally, patients will be sedated, intubated and ventilated before cardioversion. However, if shock is present, cardioversion should not be delayed, and common sense should dictate the correct sequence and timing of events.

Treatment of arrhythmias in children is complex and should be directed by a paediatric cardiologist. The discussion above merely gives a guide for their management in the emergency setting.

See chapter 9 for further discussion on the management of arrhythmias.

Stabilisation

This begins with a full assessment. Immediate resuscitation steps have been undertaken either by you or the referring team prior to your arrival. Rather than diving in sorting out lines and infusions, take time to go through the history with the senior nursing and medical staff available. This recognises their important role in the care of the child, makes sure that details recorded in the initial referring call are accurate, and brings you up to date with any changes since your last contact. Clarify any points that are unclear.

Then examine the patient. Examination will be adapted for each individual situation, and the assessment and examination of the patient following trauma are outlined in chapter 10. However, a full examination is appropriate and essential to detect those little problems (like fixed and dilated pupils) that may cause embarrassment later (Box 7.3). In an unfamiliar and stressful environment, it is easy to forget parts of the examination, and a systems approach, using the parameters outlined above in "Recognition and assessment of the sick child", is useful. In the child following trauma, treat the cervical spine as if it is damaged until investigations are normal and the child wakes up and tells you that it is not.

Box 7.3 Systems approach to examination

Respiratory system – adequacy of airway
Cardiovascular system
Neurological system
Cervical spine and trauma
Abdomen
Skin

Stabilisation of the respiratory system

Patients should be well oxygenated and ventilating appropriately prior to transfer, and in mechanically ventilated patients this should be confirmed by an arterial blood gas before departure.

In self-ventilating patients, one of the most difficult decisions to make is whether to intubate and ventilate prior to departure. If in doubt, the best course of action is to perform intubation in the controlled setting of the referring hospital, rather than being forced to do so during transport. The child can often be extubated on arrival at base, and although intubation is not without risks and, particularly in upper airways obstruction such as croup, may necessitate mechanical ventilation for a couple of days, it is safer than risking respiratory arrest on the motorway.

Intubation should be undertaken in a controlled way by the most experienced person available. In many cases this will be an anaesthetist from the referring hospital. There is no shame, and a lot to be gained, from asking for their support with a difficult airway.

Once intubated, secure the endotracheal tube well, start mechanical ventilation, and confirm tube position both by auscultation, evidence of good ventilation and oxygenation, and by radiograph. Note the size of the tube and length of insertion, and any difficulties with intubation.

Oxygen requirements are often raised during transport, possibly because of changes in ventilation–perfusion ratios due to acceleration forces. It is therefore often necessary to increase the inspired oxygen concentration a little for transfer. In aeromedical transports, oxygen requirements increase due to changes in barometric pressure. However, no assumptions should be made, and pathological causes of an increased oxygen requirement should be actively sought.

Appropriate drugs will have been given for intubation. Sedation and paralysis should normally be continued during transfer, although this will depend upon the particular clinical situation.

In most cases, pneumothoraces should be drained prior to departure. This is mandatory for aeromedical transports. Underwater seals should be replaced by Heimlich (flutter) valves.

These points are covered further in chapter 8.

Learning points
Consider the need for mechanical ventilation carefully.
Confirm endotracheal tube placement clinically and radiographically.
Secure the tube well.
Obtain satisfactory blood gases while ventilating on the transport ventilator before leaving.
Consider the need for sedation and paralysis.

Stabilisation of the cardiovascular system

Patients should be as haemodynamically stable as you can get them before departure from the referring hospital. Ideally this means having a normal heart rate, good perfusion and urine output, normal oxygen saturation and blood gas values, and a normal blood pressure.

The first step in stabilisation, after the clinical examination and any appropriate resuscitation, is to start monitoring (Box 7.4). Minimum monitoring requirements are discussed in chapter 4.

Box 7.4 Cardiovascular monitoring

ECG and heart rate
Oxygen saturation
Blood pressure (invasive or non-invasive using appropriate equipment)
Toe and core temperature
Central venous pressure where appropriate

Clinical examination and monitoring may suggest intervention such as fluid administration or inotropes as the next step. As in the intensive care unit, a good understanding of the underlying pathophysiology is essential to guide rational therapy.

In general, the physiology of transport means that patients with compensated shock will deteriorate during transfer, as fluid will tend to pool in the peripheries due to accelerational

Table 7.4 Effects of inotropic drugs (see also chapter 9)

	Heart rate	Contractility	SVR	Route	Dose
Dopamine	Increases	Increases	Increases	C	2–20
Dobutamine	Increases	Increases	Same or ↓	C/P	2–20
Epinephrine (adrenaline)	Increases	Increases	Small ↑	C	0·05–5·0
Norepinephrine (noradrenaline)	Small ↑	Small ↑	Big ↑	C	0·05–5·0
Enoximone	Mod ↑	Mod ↑	Same	C/P	5–20

SVR = systemic vascular resistance, C = central, P = peripheral. Doses are in micrograms/kg/min.

forces in the ambulance. Many patients therefore require infusion of fluid during the preparation phase.

Inotropic support may be needed (see chapter 9), particularly in the shocked patient who does not respond adequately to a fluid challenge. Although dobutamine may be given peripherally, inotrope administration will normally necessitate the placement of a central venous line, and the patient requiring inotropic support should usually have invasive arterial blood pressure monitoring as well (Table 7.4).

Patients with surgically correctable haemorrhage should have this dealt with before transfer. The transfer team may be involved in stabilising the child before and after this, prior to transfer.

Ensure that you have at least two good, working points of intravenous access. These should be well secured, and one should be easily available during the transfer for administering bolus drugs, emergency drugs and volume as required.

These points are covered further below and in chapter 9.

> *Learning points*
> Patients should be as haemodynamically stable as you can get them before departure from the referring hospital.
> Patients with compensated shock will deteriorate during transfer, so treat this before departure.
> The patient requiring inotropic support should usually have invasive arterial blood pressure monitoring in transit.
> Ensure that you have at least two good, working points of intravenous access.

Stabilisation of the central nervous system

The most common group of patients with CNS disease requiring transfer are those with traumatic head injury. This will be covered in chapter 10,

but it is worth emphasising that the priority of the transfer team is to *minimise secondary brain injury* due to hypotension and hypoxia. Thus the road traffic accident victim with a contused brain will suffer much more cerebral damage if he or she has a cardiac arrest due to the tension pneumothorax that you missed in your rush to get to the neurosurgical unit than if you had sorted this out prior to transfer.

For the patient with prolonged seizures, first ensure the patency of the airway and adequacy of ventilation. Check that there is not a biochemical cause by measuring the blood sugar and electrolytes. Follow the suggested therapeutic pathway given in Box 7.5.

> **Box 7.5** Treatment of prolonged seizures (see also chapter 13)
>
> Establish airway and oxygenation
> Diazepam 0·5mg/kg PR or lorazepam 0·1 mg/kg IV
> Commence monitoring and get IV access if not already started
> Check BM sticks, blood gas, and electrolytes
> Lorazepam 0·1 mg/kg IV
> Paraldehyde 0·4 ml/kg in arachis oil PR
> Phenytoin 20 mg/kg slow IV, with ECG monitoring
> Paralyse and ventilate, thiopentone infusion, ECG monitoring

Rarely, you will be asked to transfer a child who apparently has no hope of survival or appears to be brain dead. This difficult scenario is discussed further in chapter 12.

Stabilisation of the gastrointestinal system

Most sick children, and certainly those receiving mechanical ventilation or being transported by air, should have a nasogastric tube passed and left on free drainage. Feeds should be stopped and the stomach aspirated for the transfer to minimise the risk of vomiting and aspiration of stomach contents into the lungs.

Rarely, for long distance or prolonged transfers of stable children (particularly neonates), it may be appropriate to continue nasogastric feeds. In this case the nasogastric tube should be aspirated regularly to detect gastric stasis and prevent vomiting.

Stabilisation of the renal system

Consider urethral catheterisation in children with shock (to monitor urine output), in children who are paralysed and sedated (to prevent urinary retention), and in children who have received diuretics or mannitol (for the above reasons and also to prevent them urinating all over your equipment).

Acute hyperkalaemia

This may be due to impaired excretion (renal failure, adrenal insufficiency), increased administration (IV fluids, transfusion), and endogenous release (burns, rhabdomyolysis, haemolysis). The main clinical effect of importance to the transferring team is abnormal cardiac conduction (Box 7.6).

Treatment depends upon the underlying cause, the serum potassium level, and the presence of ECG changes (Table 7.5). If the serum potassium is

---

> **Box 7.6** ECG changes in acute hyperkalaemia
>
> Tall, peaked T waves
> Small amplitude R wave
> Small amplitude P wave
> Widened QRS
> Ventricular tachycardia
> Ventricular fibrillation

7 mmol/l or greater, or there are ECG changes, immediate therapy is necessary.

- Stop further potassium administration.
- Antagonise the cardiac conduction effects by administering calcium.
- Encourage renal excretion of potassium with furosemide (frusemide), where appropriate.
- Increase the cellular uptake of potassium by giving sodium bicarbonate or dextrose and insulin.
- Remove potassium from the body by using exchange resins.
- Treat the underlying disease.

> *Learning points*
> In patients with CNS disease, minimise secondary brain injury due to hypotension and hypoxia.
> Treatment of prolonged seizures should commence with ensuring a patent airway and oxygenation, and follow established therapeutic algorithms.
> Consider the placement of a nasogastric tube and urethral catheter prior to leaving the referring hospital.

Table 7.5 Treatment of hyperkalaemia

Drug	Dose	Onset	Duration	Comments
Calcium chloride	25 mg/kg	minutes	30 min	Give slowly IV over 5 minutes. Transient effect on ECG. If repeated doses needed, monitor serum ionised Ca^{2+}
Sodium bicarbonate	2·5 mmol/kg	< 30 min	few hours	Monitor blood pH. Beware sodium overload
Sodium chloride	25 mg/kg			Transient effect, useful if patient hyponatraemic
Dextrose + insulin	0·5 g/kg dextrose with 0·05unit/kg insulin	< 30 min	few hours	Monitor blood glucose carefully. Additional glucose may be given if BM start to fall. *Beware hypoglycaemia*
Sodium polysterene (kayexalate)	0·5–1 g/kg PO, NG, or PR	< 24 h		Note: constipation
Nebulised salbutamol	2·5–10 mg	< 30 min		

Once the patient is on the transport trolley or incubator and observations are satisfactory, the stabilisation phase finishes with a final review and checklist (Box 7.7).

Box 7.7 Predeparture checklist

1. *Airway*
   Intubation needed?
   Secure endotracheal tube?
   Position?
   Suction available?
   Oxygen for more than anticipated length of journey?

2. *Circulation*
   Adequately perfused?
   Blood pressure satisfactory?
   Ongoing circulatory losses to be considered?

3. *Temperature*
   Blankets/prewarmed incubator available?
   Ambulance heating on?
   Working temperature monitor available?

4. *Procedures*
   Reliable IV access established (preferably two IV lines *in situ*)
   Nasogastric tube (if bowel obstruction/ileus, ventilated or air transport)
   Urethral catheter (unconscious/sedated and diuretics)

5. *Monitoring*
   Check availability and function of:
   ECG
   Pulse oximeter/transcutaneous oxygen monitor
   Blood pressure monitor
   Temperature monitor
   Blood sugar monitoring

6. *Equipment*
   Is all equipment working and are the batteries charged?
   Spare batteries where possible

7. *Drugs/fluids*
   Maintenance fluid—appropriate type and rate.
   Ensure availability of:
   Emergency drugs
   Adequate sedation
   Special drugs which may be needed

Ensure that all supplies needed are available and drugs drawn up where appropriate. Talk to the parents and allow them to see the child. Thank the referring staff. Contact your base hospital advising them of your departure, the current status of the patient, and what drugs and equipment will be needed on arrival at base.

Procedures in resuscitation and stabilisation phase

This section describes some of the technical procedures in which the transporting team should be competent. The indications, limitations, and complications of each are given.

Endotracheal intubation

This is described in chapter 8.

Needle cricothyroidotomy

Indications

Inability to ventilate or oxygenate the patient by any other means.

Method

- Place the patient in the supine position.
- Locate the cricothyroid membrane by feeling for the thyroid cartilage and locating its inferior pole in the midline (Fig. 7.6).
- Extend the neck slightly if able (but not if there is any chance of a cervical spine injury).
- Take a cricothyroidotomy catheter or an 18 gauge IV catheter with a 5 ml syringe attached.
- Clean the skin over the cricothyroid membrane.
- Hold the trachea steady with one hand.
- Pass the catheter through the cricothyroid membrane at an angle of 45°, aspirating on the syringe as you go.
- When air is aspirated, the tip of the catheter is in the trachea.
- Change the angle of approach to around 20°. Advance the catheter and withdraw the needle as you would if cannulating a vein.
- Repeated aspiration of air confirms that the cannula is still in the trachea.
- Attach a Y-connector to the cannula, and attach oxygen tubing to the Y-connector.
- Set the oxygen flow rate at 1 litre per year of age of the child.
- Occlude the open end of the Y-connector for 1 second, so that oxygen passes into the trachea.
- Release the open end of the connector to allow passive exhalation (through the upper airway).
- Arrange definitive airway care.

Limitations

Insufflation of oxygen through a narrow catheter will not ventilate the patient, merely provide

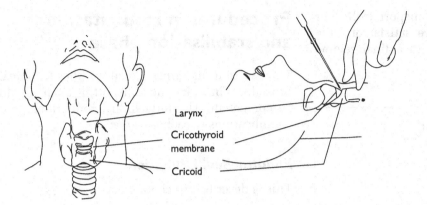

Figure 7.6 Cricothyroidotomy. (Adapted from Advanced Life Support Group. *Advanced Paediatric Life Support*, 3rd edn. London: BMJ Books, 2001.)

oxygenation, but will buy you time to get help and secure the airway in a more definitive manner (i.e. a surgical airway).

Expiration does not occur through the catheter, but passively through the upper airway. If this is *completely* blocked, and expiration does not occur at all, reduce the insufflating flow to 1–2 l/min, and get on with a definitive procedure.

When insufflating, start off at the suggested gas flow, but if there is no chest movement, increase the flow gradually.

Complications

Bleeding, false passage, surgical emphysema, damage to the surrounding tissues.

Needle thoracotomy

Indications

Suspected tension pneumothorax.

Method

- Locate the second intercostal space in the midclavicular line.
- Clean the skin over the selected area.
- Select an 18 or 20 gauge cannula or butterfly, connected to a three-way tap and syringe.
- Insert the cannula vertically through the chest, just above the third rib (to avoid the intercostal vessels and nerves).
- Aspirate as you go.
- If air is aspirated, remove the needle leaving the cannula in place.
- Drain the pneumothorax by repeated aspiration via the three-way tap.
- Insert a chest drain.

Complications

- 20% chance of causing a pneumothorax if the patient did not have one before (check with an x ray film; insert a chest drain anyway if the patient is ventilated).
- Damage to the intercostal vessels and nerves.

Chest drain insertion

Indications

To drain a pneumothorax or pleural effusion.

Method

- Select the chest drain—usually the biggest that will fit between the ribs.
- Place the patient on the unaffected side, with the uppermost arm abducted above the head.
- Locate the fifth intercostal space in the midaxillary line (usual site, others may be used in specific situations).
- Clean the skin over the selected area.
- Anaesthetise the skin with local anaesthetic.
- Make a 2 cm incision along the line of the ribs, just above the rib below the space you are aiming for (to avoid the intercostal vessels and nerves).
- Bluntly dissect the subcutaneous tissues and muscle by inserting closed forceps through the skin and opening them in the tissues.
- Dissect down to the pleura using this method (not the scalpel), and pierce this with the forceps or your finger.
- Insert the chest drain (without the trocar) through the track into the pleural space during expiration. Listen for air movement and watch for fogging inside the drain to confirm placement in the pleura.

- Normally aim the chest drain anteriorly and towards the head.
- Connect the drain to a Heimlich valve or underwater seal.
- Secure the chest drain in place.
- Take a check *x* ray film.

Limitations

The drain may become obstructed by overlying lung, or may be placed inappropriately to drain the pneumothorax. Suction applied to the chest drain may be necessary to keep up with a large air leak.

Complications

- Damage to the intercostal vessels and nerves.
- Damage to the underlying lung or viscera, including the heart and great vessels or the liver.

Never force the chest drain in with the trocar. Imagine the scene – you push with all your might, suddenly the drain goes through the intercostal tissues, there is no resistance and before you know what has happened, you have speared the heart. *Never force the chest drain in with the trocar.*

Intraosseous needle insertion

Indications

Intraosseous needles provide a rapid alternative to peripheral cannulae during resuscitation. They are effective in neonates, infants, and younger children. There is no maximum age but the technique becomes progressively less useful with increasing age. Gaining access through bone becomes more difficult, the intraosseous compartment becomes less vascular, and the limited infusion rates imposed by high resistance make it harder to deliver useful volumes of resuscitation fluid.

The main role of intraosseous access will be in the urgent resuscitation of patients to be transferred. Adequate venous access should always be subsequently established. Electing to set out on a transfer relying on intraosseous access is desperate in the extreme and should not be considered unless all other options have been excluded. Use of an intraosseous needle to gain access during the transfer usually indicates insufficient access was gained during stabilisation.

Method

- Select the appropriate site. The proximal tibia is the commonest, medial to and 1 cm below the tibial tuberosity. Other sites are shown in Figure 7.7.
- Clean the skin, infiltrate local anaesthetic if appropriate.
- Hold the leg by placing the fingers and thumb on either side.
- Hold the needle near its tip, and insert it at 90° to the skin, until a sudden loss of resistance is felt as the needle goes through the cortex of the bone.
- Confirm placement by:
  - sudden loss of resistance
  - aspirating marrow
  - needle stands proud
  - no evidence of extravasation.
- Secure the needle
- Give a bolus of fluid and drugs.

Limitations

- Specialised needles are available and should be used. Spinal needles tend to bend and ordinary needles may get blocked with bone as they have no trocar.
- A less satisfactory technique in children over 6 years (loss of marrow space). Sternum and iliac crest sites are associated with increased damage to surrounding tissues.
- Fluids and drugs need to be infused actively, as they will not flow passively by gravity.
- All commonly used resuscitation drugs and fluids can be given via the intraosseous route.
- The intraosseous needle is unstable. A method for securing it using tape and artery forceps is shown in Figure 7.8.

Complications

- Extravasation, fracture, osteomyelitis, damage to the growth plate, damage to surrounding structures.
- Missing the bone and impaling the operator (especially if the leg is not held properly).
- Despite their usefulness in resuscitation, intraosseous needles are not appropriate access with which to embark on a transfer. Needles are difficult to stabilise or secure. They are held in place largely by the bone into which they are inserted. Over time the track

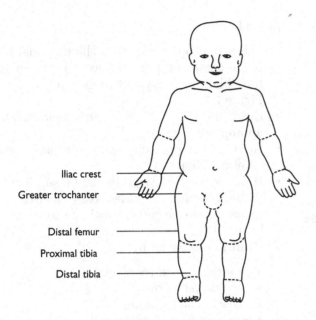

Figure 7.7 Possible sites for intraosseous needle insertion.

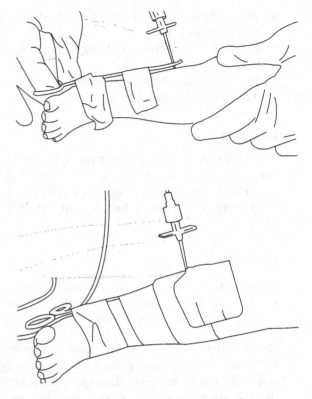

Figure 7.8 Securing the intraosseous needle.

through the bone is widened by movement of the needle and fluids or drugs administered into the needle often partially extravasate.

Central venous cannulation

Indications

- Intravenous fluid and drug administration, especially of phlebotoxic and concentrated drugs and infusions.
- Monitoring of central venous pressure.

Method

Usual sites of insertion include the femoral, internal or external jugular and subclavian veins. Long silastic catheters ("linguine lines") may also be inserted via a peripheral vein, but cannot be used for pressure monitoring.

A degree of psychomotor skill, knowledge of the anatomy, and an appreciation of the risk–benefit ratio are needed by people attempting central venous cannulation. These operator characteristics are the key to success, along with correct positioning of the patient prior to cannulation, strict asepsis, and proper fixation of the cannula once it is in.

Candidates should learn the anatomical markers for central line insertion, the details of the techniques, the complications of different approaches, and then obtain first hand experience in a controlled situation (i.e. theatre or the catheter laboratory) under supervision.

Seldinger technique (Fig. 7.9)

This is the preferred method for central venous cannulation, in which a small needle is used to locate the vessel, and a guide wire is passed through the needle, which is then removed. The larger cannula is then passed over the guide wire into the vein. The wire is removed, the cannula secured and its position confirmed by aspirating venous blood, transducing the venous pressure, and x ray film.

Femoral venous cannulation has a low rate of serious complications. The patient is positioned with the leg externally rotated and the hip slightly flexed. A roll under the buttocks may be helpful.

Local contraindications include local sepsis and intra-abdominal masses. Complications include sepsis (especially to the hip joint), and trauma to the femoral artery or nerve. If the artery is inadvertently entered too high, bleeding can occur into the retroperitoneal space, which may be impossible to control.

(a)

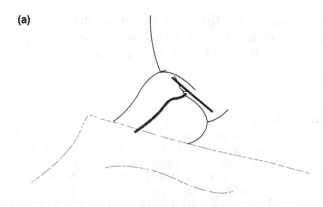

(a) Select your equipment and prepare the site. Review the anatomy. The vein lies medial to the artery, and should be cannulated 1 cm or more below the inguinal ligament.

(b)

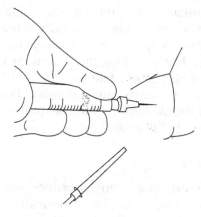

(b) Apply local anaesthetic if appropriate. Enter the skin at an angle of about 45°, aspirating as you go. Ensure the guide wire is within reach without having to turn or stretch for it.

(c)

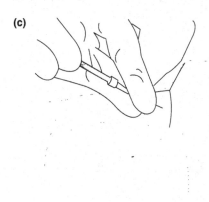

(c) When the vein is entered (flashback), hold the needle in position, remove the syringe (blood should flow back), and insert the wire. *This is the most difficult bit.* If there is *any* resistance to the wire, you are probably not in the vein—withdraw the wire, replace the syringe, and find the vein again. It is useful to have a spare wire, in case you damage the first. Make sure that it is the same length and gauge as the original. *Never lose control of the wire. You must keep hold of one end of it at all times, or risk it being lost in the patient.*

(d)

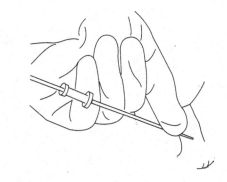

(d) Once the wire is in the vein 10–15 cm, withdraw the needle. Thread the dilator over the wire, through the skin, and into the vein. There can be some resistance to this, and it may be necessary to nick the skin with a scalpel to get the dilator through. When advancing the dilator, it is possible to kink the guide wire and follow a false passage. Occasionally move the guide wire backwards and forwards to confirm that it moves easily and that it is not kinked.

(e)

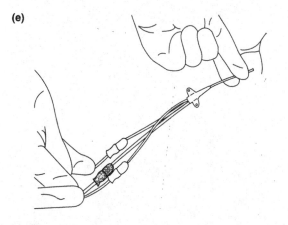

(e) Leaving the wire in the vein, remove the dilator. Have a swab ready, as the site will bleed. Keep control of the wire at all times. Thread the preflushed catheter over the wire and into the vein. Remove the wire, aspirate the catheter, and flush with saline. Secure the catheter by suturing it to the skin and place a clear dressing over the site.

Figure 7.9 a–e Example of the Seldinger technique—femoral vein.

Cannulation of the internal jugular and subclavian veins are technically more difficult and the complications are potentially more serious. The last thing that you want to do to a child in respiratory failure on a ventilator is to give him or her a pneumothorax. However, in skilled hands, these techniques provide a useful approach to the central veins.

Limitations

Various sizes and lengths of catheter are available. Infants under 10 kg should normally have 4 FG catheters inserted, older children 5 FG, and teenagers may have up to 7 FG catheters placed percutaneously.

Single, double and triple lumen catheters are available. The lumen labelled "1" is normally the one at the tip of the catheter. This is the largest lumen, and the guide wire should be passed through this lumen during insertion.

Summary

This chapter has outlined the resuscitation and stabilisation phases of the transfer.

In many cases, this phase will have been completed by the referring team, possibly following advice from the retrieval centre.

Make a full and independent assessment of the child, including reviewing the history and a structured examination.

Initiate resuscitation where appropriate.

Aim to achieve the same level of care that you would in the paediatric intensive care unit before leaving the referring hospital.

8 Management of the airway and breathing

Objectives
To understand that AIRWAY and BREATHING should not be considered in isolation.
To appreciate the need for a low threshold for intubation and ventilation for transportation, as transportation is often associated with clinical deterioration in airway and breathing.
To understand that problems should be anticipated and prevented, and that stability must be achieved prior to embarking on transportation.

Introduction

Airway and breathing problems may be the primary reason for transportation to the paediatric or neonatal intensive care units (PICU or NICU). However, they should never be viewed in isolation, but in the context of the whole clinical picture. The management of airway and breathing is technically difficult and is the source of many adverse events occurring during transportation. Meticulous preparation and stabilisation of the child before departure minimises risk during transportation. A systematic "ABC" approach including assessment, optimisation and preparation for transportation of the airway and breathing is recommended. During transportation, airway and breathing must be regularly reassessed to evaluate the impact of treatment and recognise further deterioration, which can be rapid.

Developmental changes in airway and breathing anatomy and physiology

It is important to have an understanding of the changes in airway and breathing anatomy and physiology which occur with age. The anatomy of the neonatal and infant airway causes a predisposition to airway obstruction and high airway resistance, and can increase the difficulty of intubation (Table 8.1). The neonate and infant also have a limited respiratory reserve as a result

Table 8.1 Neonatal and infant airway and breathing anatomy

Anatomy	Effect on airway/breathing
Large occiput*	Increases neck flexion and airway obstruction
Small nares	Increases airway resistance (nasal breathers ≤ 3 months)
Large tongue*	Increases airway resistance
Low pharyngeal muscle tone	Airway obstruction by tongue
Floppy epiglottis*	Increases airway obstruction
Larynx anterior/cephalad*	
Short trachéa*	
Trachea angled posteriorly*	
Cricoid cartilage	Narrowest point up to 8 years—uncuffed tracheal tubes
Narrow airways	Increases airway resistance
Compliant airways	Collapse with increased respiratory effort
Compliant chest wall	Indrawing with increased respiratory effort
Barrel shaped chest	Horizontal ribs contribute less to breathing
Flattened diaphragm	Reduced diaphragmatic movement
Immature respiratory muscles	Reduced effectiveness of forced expiration, for example, cough

*Increases difficulty or complications of intubation.

Table 8.2 Developmental changes in airway and breathing physiology

	Neonate	Infant	Child
Respiratory rate (per min)	32	25	16
Tidal volume (ml/kg)	7	7	7
Dead space (ml/kg)	2·5	2·5	2·5
Minute volume (ml/kg/min)	224	175	112
Vital capacity (ml/kg)	40	50	60
Functional residual capacity (ml/kg)	25	30	40
O_2 consumption (ml/kg/min)	7	5	3

of the higher ratio of minute ventilation to functional residual capacity (the volume of gas in the lung at the end of tidal expiration, which acts as a reservoir of oxygen), higher closing volumes (the volume of gas in the lung at which airways in dependent areas of the lung begin to close during expiration), and higher oxygen consumption (Table 8.2). Therefore, respiratory decompensation in neonates and infants can be rapid.

Assessment of airway and breathing

Respiratory failure accounts for over 50% of PICU/NICU transfers. The majority of cases are due to primary respiratory disorders. However, respiratory failure can be caused by other organ system dysfunction including CNS, renal and metabolic conditions, and patients in haemo-dynamic shock who require airway and breathing support to decrease the work of breathing. Therefore, airway and breathing should be systematically assessed in the context of the full clinical picture. Areas to focus on are as follows.

History

- Signs and symptoms, presenting diagnosis
- Speed of deterioration
- Ongoing treatment
- Duration of intubation/previous intubation/ intubation difficulty/tracheal tube changes
- Volume of secretions/suction requirement

Examination

- Airway patency
  - "See-saw" breathing/stridor/secretions/ trauma/swelling

  - Tracheal tube—size/length/patency/position/ fixation.
- Adequacy of breathing
  - Oxygen requirement
  - Rate (trend)/cyanosis/air entry
  - Intercostals/accessory muscles
  - Chest trauma—ribs/pneumothorax/chest drain
- Level of consciousness
  - Hypoxia/hypercarbia/CNS dysfunction
- Degree of exhaustion
  - Apparent decrease in distress with deteriorating ABG.
- Sedation and neuromuscular blockade

Monitoring

- Pulse oximetry/capnography/ECG/airway pressures/Fio_2

Investigations

- ABG
- CXR
  - Tracheal tube position/lung fields/ pneumothorax

Airway and breathing should be reassessed regularly, especially after moving the patient. Immediately after changing the oxygen source of a ventilator confirm the presence of chest movement, a capnography trace if available and the pressure measured on the ventilator pressure gauge.

It is important with premature neonates to avoid hyperoxia which is associated with retinopathy of prematurity. If a patent ductus arteriosus is present be aware of the difference between preductal O_2

Box 8.1 Indications for intubation

This is a "physiological" approach rather than a long list of diagnoses, and is not exhaustive. Due to the marked differences between neonates and older children the specific values given for the respiratory and haemodynamic variables are not absolute and should act as a guide only. Specific neonatal factors are indicated in bold.

Deteriorating airway
- Chest wall recession, tracheal tug
- "See-saw" breathing
- Stridor

Respiratory distress
- Rate > 60 min
- Chest wall recession, **grunting**
- Sao_2 < 94% **(< 90% preterm)** or Pao_2 < 8 kPa **(< 6·5 kPa preterm)**
- $Paco_2$ > 6 or < 3·5 kPa
- **Recurrent apnoeas**
- Exhaustion

Shock
- HR > 180/min or < 80/min (< 5yr), > 160/min or < 60/min (> 5yr)
- Absent peripheral pulses
- Cold peripheries
- Capillary refill > 2 seconds
- Systolic blood pressure < 70 + (age in years × 2) mmHg
- **Mean blood pressure < (postconceptual age in weeks) mmHg**

Less than 30 weeks' gestation

Deteriorating level of consciousness

Recurrent seizures

---

saturation, measured from the right hand or ear lobe, and postductal O_2 saturation. The former reflects the saturation of blood delivered to the head, brain, and eyes, whereas the latter reflects the saturation of blood flowing to the rest of the body. When there is right to left shunting through the duct the preductal saturations may be significantly higher than the postductal saturations.

Deciding to intubate

Airway and breathing must be reliable before transportation. The decision to intubate can be difficult. There should be a lower threshold for intubation and ventilation for transportation than in routine PICU/NICU practice, with the aim of optimising the clinical condition before transportation (Box 8.1). Care should be taken that intubation to secure the airway or facilitate ventilation for transportation should not be perceived by the referring staff or parents as implying either inadequate prior management or deterioration in the condition of the patient

per se. Consider the entire clinical picture and discuss the decision with the supervising PICU/NICU consultant.

Intubation

Safe intubation requires an appropriately trained team, adequate preparation, and a calm methodical approach. A trained assistant is vital to apply cricoid pressure correctly, assist with the intubation technique, and administer drugs as necessary. The skills are best acquired in the operating theatre under the supervision of an experienced anaesthetist. Points worth emphasising include correct head and neck positioning to produce a direct line of sight from the mouth to the larynx. The sniffing position, with the head slightly extended on the neck and the neck slightly flexed on the trunk, is recommended (Fig. 8.1). Excessive extension or flexion will impede intubation. Patients with suspected cervical spine injury must not be positioned in this manner. The head and neck must be immobilised in the neutral position by manual in-line stabilisation during intubation.

Neonate and infant

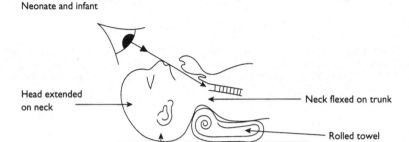

Head extended on neck

Neck flexed on trunk

Rolled towel

Large occiput

Child

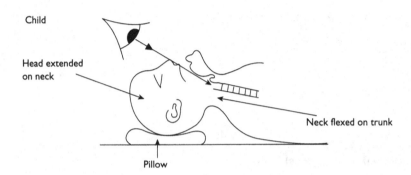

Head extended on neck

Neck flexed on trunk

Pillow

Figure 8.1 Correct head and neck position for intubation.

Preoxygenation to replace the nitrogen in the functional residual capacity of the lungs with oxygen is important to create a reservoir of oxygen to cover the apnoeic period during intubation. This is very important for neonates and infants who quickly desaturate and become hypoxic following the onset of apnoea because of high oxygen consumption and a small functional residual capacity. Bag-valve-mask apparatus is relatively simple to use, can deliver 100% oxygen (with appropriate oxygen flow and a reservoir bag, refer to the manufacturers' instructions), and can function in an emergency without an oxygen supply to ventilate the patient with ambient air. An anaesthetic "T" piece circuit (Mapleson F system) can also deliver 100% oxygen and will provide a visual clue that there is an adequate seal between the face mask and the face of the patient and it will also give information about the chest compliance and airways' resistance of the patient. It is ideal for preoxygenation of the spontaneously breathing patient, delivering 100% oxygen, if desired, with variable CPAP (continuous positive airway pressure). However, significant expertise is required for correct use. Both systems can be used with an O_2/air mixture to avoid hyperoxia in premature neonates.

Beyond the neonatal period adequate anaesthesia and neuromuscular blockade with rapidly acting drugs are essential to limit the apnoeic period. The choice of anaesthetic agent and dose requires considerable clinical experience and is largely determined by the diagnosis and haemodynamic status of the patient and the experience of the clinician. The dose ranges given in this chapter can act only as a rough guide (Table 8.3). It is uncommon for neonates to undergo a formal rapid sequence induction. Opioid sedation, with or without neuromuscular blockade, is commonly used. Awake intubation, without the use of anaesthesia or sedation, is no longer recommended except during resuscitation. It increases the risk of airway trauma, laryngospasm, and hypoxia, and causes marked tachycardia, hypertension and the possibility of intraventricular haemorrhage in premature neonates.

Cricoid pressure is a technique which is used to reduce the risk of passive regurgitation of gastric contents which may be aspirated, and helps improve the view of the larynx during laryngoscopy in neonates and infants. Pressure is applied by the assistant with two or three fingers directly down onto the cricoid cartilage, which is pushed backwards, occluding the oesophagus on the vertebral column. Cricoid pressure is applied from induction of anaesthesia and discontinued after correct placement of the tracheal tube. Incorrectly applied cricoid pressure is both

Table 8.3 Intubation drugs

Drug	Dose (mg/kg)	Onset (min)	Duration (min)
Anaesthetic drugs			
Ketamine	2	< 1	10–15
Thiopentone	3–5	< 1	5–10
Propofol	2–4	< 1	3–8
Neuromuscular blockers			
Suxamethonium	1–2	< 1	3–5
Vecuronium	0·1–0·2	1–3	20–40
Rocuronium	0·5–1·0	1–1·5	20–40
Sedative drugs			
Midazolam	0·05–0·2	2–5	30–120
Morphine	0·05–0·2	2–5	60–240
Adjunctive drugs			
Fentanyl	0·001–0·005	1–3	20–60

See chapter 13 for details of side effects and contraindications.

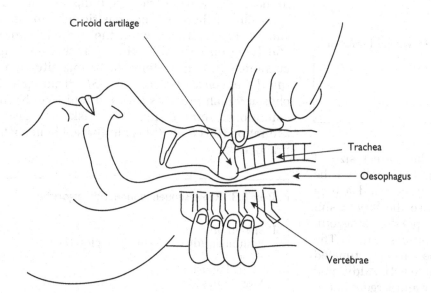

Figure 8.2 Application of two-handed cricoid pressure.

ineffective in preventing regurgitation and also distorts the larynx, significantly increasing the difficulty of intubation. If application of cricoid pressure causes excessive flexion of the head on the neck, a two-handed technique can be used with the other hand placed behind the neck of the patient to counterbalance the force and maintain the optimal position of the head and neck (Fig. 8.2).

Correct tracheal tube placement must be confirmed by observing it pass through the vocal cords, inspection and auscultation for bilateral chest movement and air entry, confirmation of end tidal CO_2 by capnography, if available, and maintenance of adequate oxygenation saturation following intubation. If in doubt about the tracheal tube placement TAKE IT OUT and recommence bag and mask ventilation.

Laryngoscopy and intubation have a number of potential adverse consequences (Box 8.2).

It is debatable whether oral or nasal intubation is preferable for transportation. Oral intubation is quicker to perform, is arguably more simple for inexperienced or infrequent practitioners, and avoids the possibility of nasal trauma and bleeding obscuring the view of the larynx during intubation. However, nasal tracheal tubes are probably more easy to secure, are less prone to movement in the trachea during tracheal suctioning, thus reducing tracheal trauma, and probably kink less during transport. Whatever route is chosen, the operator should be familiar with the technique and on completion the tube should be secure, patent, and correctly positioned.

Box 8.2 Complications of intubation

Hypoxia:
  Prolonged apnoea with inadequate
    preoxygenation
  Oesophageal intubation
  Right main bronchus intubation

Haemodynamic:
  Tachycardia
  Hypertension
  Intraventricular haemorrhage
  Bradycardia

Trauma:
  Teeth, lips, tongue, pharynx, larynx and trachea

Airway:
  Laryngospasm
  Bronchospasm
  Aspiration

It is important to choose the correct size of tracheal tube. A tube which is too small will be inadequate for ventilation in transit and a tube that is too large will traumatise the larynx and trachea, leading to swelling and possibly long term complications such as subglottic stenosis. The correct size of a tracheal tube can be estimated from the age of the patient (Table 8.4). Additional tracheal tubes one size smaller and larger should be readily available. In children younger than 8 years of age the circular cricoid cartilage is the narrowest part of the airway, therefore an adequate seal can be achieved for positive pressure ventilation with an uncuffed tracheal tube. However, in children over 8 years of age the airway is narrowest at the vocal cords, therefore a cuffed tracheal tube is required to make a seal within the trachea for ventilation. The trachea of neonates and infants is relatively short and the position of the head can significantly alter the position of the tube in the trachea. Therefore, it is important to estimate the required length of the tracheal tube from the age of the patient (Table 8.4) and confirm correct positioning on chest radiograph. The use of tracheal tubes

smaller than 2·5 mm is not recommended as they are virtually impossible to suction through and therefore dangerous during transportation.

Effective tracheal tube fixation is essential for transportation. The tracheal tube may be tied, taped, or fixed with dedicated tube fixators. The tracheal tube position and length should be rechecked after fixation. Intubated children should be given sedative and neuromuscular blocking drugs throughout transportation to reduce the likelihood of accidental extubation. However, premature neonates often only require sedation for transportation.

Special considerations

The full stomach

An acutely ill or injured child should be assumed to have delayed gastric emptying and a "full stomach". If there is a nasogastric tube *in situ* it should be aspirated with the patient supine and lying on each side. However, this does not guarantee an empty stomach. In this situation a *rapid sequence induction (RSI)* technique is chosen which provides safe and rapid intubating conditions, minimising the risk of gastric aspiration (Box 8.3). RSI is rarely used in neonatal practice.

Box 8.3 Rapid sequence induction algorithm

Preparation:
  Equipment/drugs (+ emergency)/patient
  IV access
  Skilled assistant
  Monitoring
  Aspirate nasogastric tube
  Yankuer suction
  Tipping bed/cot

Preoxygenation
Administer anaesthetic agent
Cricoid pressure
Administer suxamethonium
Intubation
Position check
Tracheal tube fixation
Position check

RSI requires thorough preparation and effective teamwork. The aim is to minimise the time from administration of the anaesthetic induction agent, which will result in the loss of the protective airway reflexes, to correct placement of the

Table 8.4 Tracheal tube sizes

Tracheal tube size	Age of infant
Internal diameter (mm)	
2·5–3·0	Premature neonate
3·0	Term neonate
3·5	6 months
4·0	I year
(Age/4) +4	> I year
Length (cm)	
3 × internal diameter oral, add 3 cm for nasal	< I year
(Age/2) +12 oral, add 3 cm for nasal	> I year

Note: detailed sizes for oral and nasal neonatal tracheal tubes are given in Appendix 2.

tracheal tube by using rapidly acting anaesthetic drugs. Other safety measures include cricoid pressure to reduce the risk of passive regurgitation of gastric contents and preoxygenation to prevent hypoxia during the apnoeic period. Ketamine, thiopentone or propofol are suitable agents for induction of anaesthesia (Table 8.3). However, benzodiazepines such as midazolam cannot be recommended in this situation because of a slow onset of action. Suxamethonium is the neuromuscular blocking drug of choice because of its rapid onset of action, producing optimal intubating conditions within 30–45 seconds. An additional benefit of suxamethonium is its short duration of action of 3–5 minutes in the majority of patients. Patients who prove to be un-intubatable hopefully will resume spontaneous breathing before the preoxygenation reserve in the functional residual capacity of the lungs is exhausted and hypoxia develops. This is in contrast to the non-depolarising neuromuscular blockers (for example, rocuronium, atracurium, and vecuronium), which have slower onset times and considerably longer durations of action.

Airway obstruction

A gas induction should be used when there is doubt about the ability to intubate or ventilate using a bag and mask after the onset of anaesthesia and neuromuscular blockade, the classic example being epiglottitis. The aim of gas induction is gradual progression to intubating conditions, maintaining spontaneous breathing and control of the airway at all times. A gas induction should only be undertaken by a clinician with specialist anaesthetic training. If

necessary request the help of a local experienced anaesthetist or intensive care clinician.

The difficult airway

The most common cause of difficulty with intubation for the inexperienced or infrequent practitioner is poor technique (Box 8.4). If intubation is not achieved rapidly, attempts should cease and bag and mask ventilation be recommenced. The head and neck positioning is reviewed prior to a possible further attempt being made. However, excessive attempts at intubation should not be undertaken. The primary concern is the maintenance of adequate oxygenation by bag and mask ventilation (Box 8.5). If necessary the patient should be woken up and a more experienced clinician summoned for further

---

Box 8.4 Common technical reasons for difficulty in intubation

Head and neck position:
  Overextension of the head on the neck
  Inadequate flexion of the neck on the trunk

Laryngoscopy:
  Failure to sweep the tongue to the left side of the mouth
  Leverage of the laryngoscope instead of lifting along the axis of the laryngoscope handle

Obstruction of the view:
  Tracheal tube or operator's hand in the line of sight
  Inadequate suctioning of secretions

Inadequate anaesthesia or neuromuscular blockade

Box 8.5 Failed intubation drill

Maintenance of oxygenation is the priority
Call for HELP
Do not make persistent attempts at intubation
Do not give repeated doses of neuromuscular
blocking drugs
Maintain a patent airway
Bag and mask ventilate to maintain oxygenation
Continue cricoid pressure unless it is impeding
ventilation
Turn onto left side and place head down unless
this impedes ventilation

---

attempts at intubation. A difficult airway can also
result from a variety of anatomical problems, and
these should be excluded during the initial
patient assessment (Boxes 8.6, 8.7). Careful choice
of tracheal tube size, laryngoscope blade and the
availability of adjuncts (for example, stylets and
bougies) are important. If in doubt, summon

Box 8.6 Common anatomical reasons for
difficulty with intubation

Limited access to the oropharynx:
    Facial trauma

Obstructed view of the larynx:
    Large tongue
    Laryngeal tumour/papillomata
    Short mandible (Pierre Robin)
    Epiglottitis

Narrow larynx:
    Croup

Narrow trachea:
    Subglottic stenosis
    Tracheal web

Box 8.7 Preintubation assessment

History:
    Current illness
    Previous intubation details
    Predisposing diagnoses, for example Pierre Robin

Examination:
    Head—shape/size
    Mouth—size/opening
    Teeth—size/integrity
    Mandible—size/receding
    Tongue—size
    Neck—mobility/cervical spine injury/swelling/
        masses

---

experienced help for consideration of gas
induction or fibreoptic intubation. It is vitally
important during attempted intubation that the
scenario of *"can't intubate, can't ventilate"* is
avoided.

Shock

A significant percentage of cardiac output is
delivered to the respiratory muscles of shocked
patients. Positive pressure ventilation reduces
this and diverts blood flow to the vital organs.
However, anaesthetic agents used for intubation
can cause a significant drop in cardiac output and
blood pressure and must be used cautiously.

Raised intracranial pressure

Patients with raised intracranial pressure require
intubation and controlled hyperventilation
for both airway protection and to decrease
intracranial pressure. Adequate anaesthesia is
required to prevent an acute rise in intracranial
pressure caused by the haemodynamic response
to laryngoscopy and intubation. A dose of opioid
(for example, fentanyl) is recommended as an
adjunct to the anaesthetic agent to blunt this
unwanted response. Ketamine is specifically
contraindicated as it causes a rise in intracranial
pressure.

Key points for intubation
Oxygenation is always the priority.
Never lose control of the airway.
Bag-valve-mask ventilation is the default position of
    safety.
An adequately trained team (intubator and assistant)
    is required/ask for help.
Adequate patient assessment and equipment
    preparation.
Plan for a failed intubation.

Mechanical ventilation

A selection of portable, gas driven mechanical
ventilators is required to deliver the range of tidal
volumes required for neonates and children of all
ages. Ideally they should have disconnection and
high pressure alarms and variable respiratory rate,
peak inspiratory pressure, tidal volume, Fio_2,
I : E ratio, and PEEP (positive end expiratory
pressure). A controlled or mandatory ventilation
mode, either "pressure control" or "volume
control", is recommended for transportation. The

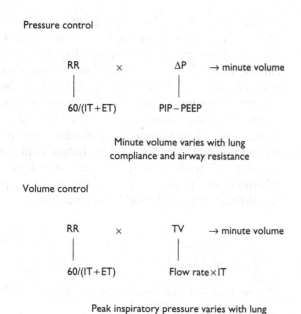

Pressure control

$$RR \quad \times \quad \Delta P \quad \rightarrow \text{minute volume}$$

$$60/(IT+ET) \qquad PIP-PEEP$$

Minute volume varies with lung
compliance and airway resistance

Volume control

$$RR \quad \times \quad TV \quad \rightarrow \text{minute volume}$$

$$60/(IT+ET) \qquad \text{Flow rate} \times IT$$

Peak inspiratory pressure varies with lung
compliance and airway resistance

Figure 8.3 Ventilator settings. RR = respiratory rate,
ΔP = change in airway pressure on inspiration,
PIP = peak inspiratory pressure, PEEP = positive end
expiratory pressure, IT = inspiratory time, ET = expiratory
time, TV = tidal volume.

patient's intrinsic respiratory effort is suppressed by sedation with or without neuromuscular blockade. "Pressure control" is recommended for neonates, infants and young children for several reasons. Minute ventilation is more predictable when using uncuffed tracheal tubes with an obligatory inspiratory leak. The risk of barotrauma is reduced if sedation and neuromuscular blockade are inadequate and the patient "fights" the ventilator. In "pressure control" ventilation the peak inspiratory pressure is set on the ventilator and the delivered tidal volume will depend on the patient's airway resistance and lung compliance. The tidal volume will be reduced by high airway resistance (for example, asthma) and by low lung compliance (for example, adult respiratory distress syndrome (ARDS)). In "volume control" the tidal volume is set directly or indirectly by setting the inspiratory time and inspiratory flow rate and the peak inspiratory pressure is dependent on the lung compliance. It is ideally used in conjunction with a cuffed tracheal tube with no inspiratory leak, which is usually reserved for children over 8 years of age. "Volume control" ventilation is useful when close control of minute volume and CO_2 is required (for example, raised intracranial

pressure). However, there is a risk of barotrauma unless an upper pressure limit is set appropriately. In practice, the currently available "pressure control" transport ventilators (for example, babyPAC, SIMS pneuPAC) will cope easily with neonates and infants up to 10 kg. Bigger children will require to be ventilated using a "volume control" ventilator (for example, ventiPAC, SIMS pneuPAC). However, for children less than 8 years of age with uncuffed tracheal tubes and an obligatory inspiratory leak, the "volume control" ventilator is set up in a fashion to simulate many aspects of "pressure control" ventilation. Fio_2, respiratory rate and I : E ratio are set as for "pressure control" (Fig. 8.3). However, the inspiratory flow on the "volume control" ventilator is increased from a low level to achieve the desired chest expansion and peak inspiratory pressure on the ventilator pressure gauge. With this technique it is important to set the peak inspiratory pressure limit to just above this level to protect from barotrauma and to give an early warning of changing conditions, for example tracheal tube blockage or inadequate sedation and neuromuscular blockade. Transport ventilators are, by design, less sophisticated than their intensive care counterparts. Therefore, it can be difficult to achieve a comparable Pao_2 and $Paco_2$ in transit. It is advisable to establish the patient on the transport ventilator as early as possible to allow adequate time to manipulate the ventilator settings, including the use of PEEP to optimise the blood gases before transportation.

Patient packaging

Children intubated with an uncuffed tracheal tube require a nasogastric tube to avoid gaseous gastric distension. Pneumothoraces should be drained before departure because positive pressure ventilation or flying at altitude can cause them to expand, resulting in respiratory and cardiovascular compromise. One-way flutter (Heimlich) valves may be used in preference to bottles with underwater seals for chest drains during transportation. The child's head and tracheal and ventilator tubes should be securely fixed whilst ensuring easy access for airway management. Emergency drugs, airway and ventilation equipment (including a self-inflating resuscitation bag, valve and mask system) must be immediately available. A predeparture checklist prevents accidental omissions in stabilisation.

Adverse events in transit

Problems which have been reported in transit with airway and breathing include hypoxia, tracheal tube blockage, accidental tracheal extubation, ventilator malfunction, and exhaustion of the oxygen supply. During transportation the child should be regularly reassessed using a systematic ABC approach. The position, patency and fixation of the tracheal tube are confirmed. Capnography is a sensitive way of monitoring airway security in the intubated child, especially during periods of maximal risk such as loading and unloading from vehicles when clinical observation is difficult. In transit, there is a significant risk of tracheal tube blockage by secretions, which can be reduced by humidifying the inspired gas using a heat and moisture exchanging filter (HME) and by regular tracheal suction. Adequacy of ventilation is assessed by observing chest movement, the airway pressure gauge on the ventilator, and the capnograph trace. The ventilator settings, connections and oxygen source are regularly observed. The well known mnemonic, DOPE, is a useful method of troubleshooting clinical deterioration (consider Displacement or Obstruction of the tracheal tube, Pneumothorax and Equipment problems). Intubated patients require sedation and usually neuromuscular blockade for transportation to reduce the possibility of accidental extubation, decrease awareness and anxiety, and facilitate controlled ventilation with the transport ventilator. If reintubation is necessary in transit, transport should be temporarily halted if possible.

Summary
AIRWAY and BREATHING should not be considered in isolation.
A low threshold for intubation and ventilation for transportation is needed.
Transportation is often associated with clinical deterioration in airway and breathing.
Problems should be anticipated and prevented.
Stability must be achieved prior to embarking on transportation.

9   Management of the circulation

Objectives
Discussion of the management of the circulation in the transport environment covering: physiology; assessment; monitoring; stabilisation; and congenital cardiac disease.

Introduction

The circulation is the body's system for transporting oxygen, and other essential substrates, to its tissues and organs. The overall function of the circulation is dependent on multiple factors with the heart, the circulating volume of blood, and the integrity of the blood vessels all contributing.

Maintaining a stable circulation is fundamental to intensive care and therefore the transfer of intensive care patients. In the transport environment this can be particularly difficult but no less important. Failure to achieve this stability endangers the patient in the short term and can have profound long term consequences.

Physiology

The principal function of the circulation is to distribute oxygen and other essential supplies to the tissues and organs of the body. Understanding the circulation in this way makes it easier to understand how it goes wrong and what to do about it.

Oxygen carriage and delivery

Oxygen in the blood is mainly carried by the haemoglobin in red blood cells. A small amount is dissolved in the plasma but this is generally so small as to be insignificant. "Oxygen saturation" is the percentage of haemoglobin that is carrying oxygen.

$$\text{Oxygen content in blood} = \text{Hb} \times \text{oxygen saturation}$$

As excessively high haemoglobin concentration makes the blood too viscous to pump, efficient oxygen delivery depends on a normal haemoglobin concentration and good oxygenation. When this has been achieved the amount of oxygen delivered to the tissues will be determined by how much blood the heart pumps, i.e. the cardiac output.

$$\text{Oxygen delivery} = \text{oxygen content} \times \text{cardiac output}$$

Cardiac output

The amount of blood pumped into the circulation by the heart is the cardiac output. This is adjusted by a variety of control mechanisms to meet the body's demand for oxygen and to maintain an adequate blood pressure (Table 9.1). It increases to meet the demands associated with muscle activity, heat production, or illness. The cardiac output may be unable to meet the metabolic demands of the body because the heart's ability to pump blood decreases, the need increases, or a combination of both. Any situation where the cardiac output is insufficient for the body's needs is called "shock".

Cardiac output is determined by how much blood is pumped by each contraction (stroke

Table 9.1 Normal cardiovascular values

	30 weeks' gestation newborn	< 1 year	2–5 years	5–12 years	> 12 years
Heart rate maximum/min	170	160	140	120	100
Heart rate minimum/min	120	110	95	80	60
Systolic blood pressure (lowest normal) mmHg	50	70	80	90	100
Mean blood pressure (lowest normal) mmHg	30	50	55	65	70

Notes: O_2 demand = 3–7 ml/kg/min, arterial O_2 content = $((\text{Hb}) \times 1 \cdot 34) + (0 \cdot 003 \times Pao_2)$ ml/dl, intravascular volume = 75–80 ml/kg.

volume) and how often the heart contracts (heart rate).

$$\text{Cardiac output} = \text{stroke volume} \times \text{heart rate}$$

Stroke volume is determined by how well the ventricle fills between beats and its ability to pump the blood forward when it contracts.

The most important factor in ventricular filling is the volume of blood in the circulation. As the volume of blood increases the venous pressure rises and more blood flows into the ventricles between contractions. Stroke volume increases as venous pressure increases until the ventricle becomes overdistended. Overdistension of the ventricle impairs its ability to contract and the stroke volume decreases again.

Young, and especially premature infants, are less able to vary their stroke volume than older children and adults, and are therefore more dependent on heart rate changes to vary their cardiac output.

Blood pressure

The systolic blood pressure is the maximum pressure generated in the circulation as the heart contracts. Diastolic blood pressure is the pressure maintained in the system between heart beats. Mean blood pressure is the average pressure through a cycle of systole and diastole.

Even with a low cardiac output the blood pressure can be kept high by increasing the vascular resistance. The blood flow to each organ and tissue will depend on both the cardiac output and the resistance presented by the arteries supplying that organ. The blood pressure itself does not indicate how good the flow is.

Blood flow to the heart muscle is different from the rest of the body. During contraction (systole) the pressure in the heart muscle is the same as the blood that it is pumping. This means it cannot pump blood to itself during systole. Blood flow to the heart occurs entirely during diastole and is dependent on diastolic blood pressure. In other organs the blood flow is determined by the mean blood pressure.

Blood pressure and the brain

The brain controls the blood flow it receives through a process of "autoregulation". This allows the brain to control its own blood supply regardless of what is happening to the rest of the

body—a very sensible design feature. Adequate blood flow should be maintained if the blood pressure is low, excessive flow should be prevented if the blood pressure is high.

This control system functions poorly in critically ill neonates, extremely premature infants, and patients who have suffered a traumatic or an ischaemic brain injury. In these patients the blood supply to the brain becomes dependent on blood pressure. Variations in blood pressure cause variations in blood flow to the brain. Low or variable blood pressure can cause brain ischaemia or haemorrhage.

In older children brain swelling following any type of brain injury causes a rise in intracranial pressure. This reduces the blood flow to the brain. Maintaining a high blood pressure can be necessary to provide an adequate blood flow.

Low or unstable blood pressure can result in a poor neurological outcome for:

- Extremely premature infants
- Critically ill neonates
- Infants and children with hypoxic ischaemic encephalopathy
- Children who have suffered a severe head injury

Changes in the cardiovascular system with age

The heart chambers and valves form early in fetal life but the function of the whole cardiovascular system continues to develop rapidly in the several months after birth. Development continues more slowly throughout childhood. During this time the structure of the heart changes, contractile elements in muscle increase and become more sensitive to catecholamines (for example, epinephrine). The most dramatic changes occur around the time of birth.

In utero blood is oxygenated in the placenta and the lungs have a high vascular resistance with consequently little pulmonary blood flow. Blood bypasses the lungs by flowing straight from the right to the left atrium through the foramen ovale, or by flowing from the pulmonary artery into the aorta through the ductus arteriosus (Fig. 9.1).

At birth vascular resistance in the lungs drops to allow blood to flow through them. Flow through the foramen ovale ceases. Flow through the ductus arteriosus diminishes as pressure in the pulmonary artery decreases. The ductus narrows in response to increased levels of oxygen

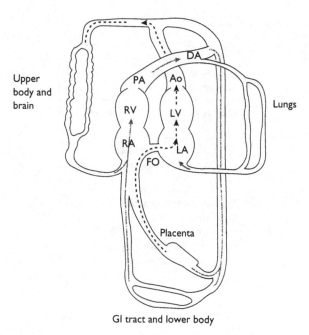

Figure 9.1 The fetal circulation. (Dr D Thomas: reproduced with permission.) PA = pulmonary artery, DA = ductus arteriosus, Ao = aorta, RV = right ventricle, LV = left ventricle, RA = right atrium, LA = left atrium, FO = foramen ovale

in the blood and usually closes within the first few days of life. Resistance in the lungs remains quite high initially then decreases over a period of months (Table 9.2).

Failure to establish adequate blood flow through the lungs at birth results in general hypoxia. Congenital structural abnormalities of the heart and major blood vessels can also prevent successful transition to a functioning cardiovascular system after birth. This is discussed below (Table 9.3).

Assessment and monitoring

Accurate assessment of the cardiovascular system is an essential part of the preparation to transfer any unwell child from one location to another. Failure to recognise a problem, or the severity of the problem, will result in inadequate stabilisation and a high chance of deterioration during the transfer. Effective intervention will be more difficult because of the limitations of the transport environment and because the problem will be more established and serious.

Inevitably some patients will deteriorate during transfer. With motion, noise, distraction, little space and a limited view of the patient it is clear that monitoring at least as comprehensive as in

the intensive care unit is necessary to detect problems.

Immediate assessment

Any patient requiring transfer should be assessed by the transferring staff as soon as possible. The most immediate assessment will be of the ABC type discussed in chapters 6 and 7.

History

Key aspects in the history should be sought while assessing the cardiovascular system.

In the newborn a history of maternal infection, peripartum haemorrhage, cardiotocograph (CTG) abnormalities, details of cord clamping, and condition at birth may indicate risk of cardiac dysfunction. The timing of the onset of illness in relation to birth will help diagnose the disease process and its likely progress.

The presentation of infants in shock, having been well at birth, within the first few days of life frequently indicates the presence of congenital cardiac disease.

In septicaemic patients a history of rapid onset and progressive deterioration is likely to indicate a need for escalating support. Stability may be difficult to achieve before transfer.

The history of the mechanism of injury in trauma patients is crucial to their assessment. In children blunt trauma to the trunk is often associated with occult damage to viscera and subsequent progressive blood loss. A history of a forceful blow should prompt careful attention to haemodynamic monitoring and venous access in children who initially seem to have only minor injuries.

The treatment the patient has received already is an important part of the history. Trends in heart rate, respiratory rate and blood pressure are valuable in assessment of the cardiovascular system. The amount of fluid that has been given and its effect on observations should be noted. The effect of drugs on the circulation should be noted, especially inotropes, diuretics, and prostaglandins.

Examination

A full clinical examination should always be made but is often neglected in intensive care environments. The orientation and emphasis of the examination will depend upon the clinical circumstances.

Table 9.2 Physiological changes from fetal to adult circulation

Effect	Mechanism
Fall in pulmonary vascular resistance and hence right ventricular force	Lung fluid emptied Air entrained
Ductus arteriosus closes functionally then anatomically	Ductus exposed to increased Pa_{O_2}
Foramen ovale functionally then anatomically shut	Right atrial and ventricular pressure below equivalents on left
Shift of dominance from right to left ventricle	Pulmonary and systemic circulations become separate Left ventricle solely responsible for systemic cardiac output

Table 9.3 Features of the newborn myocardium

At birth	Consequences	Practical considerations
Myocytes short	Relatively fixed contractility	Beware of volume overload
Paucity of contractile elements	Cardiac output rate dependent	
Activation immature	Myocardium sensitive to afterload	Avoid increasing peripheral vascular resistance
Metabolically adapted to hypoxaemia	More robust with changes in Pa_{O_2} and pH	
Parasympathetic innervation complete	Bradycardia more easily elicited with vagal stimulation	Give atropine to block vagus if stimulation anticipated
Sympathetic innervation incomplete of both heart and vasculature	Different response of vasculature to sepsis	
Ventricles of similar shape	Failure of contractility leads to biventricular failure	Assume biventricular failure in youngest children

General

Look for dysmorphic features that may be associated with particular cardiac lesions. The presence of chest scars may suggest previous cardiac surgery.

Heart rate

Tachycardia or any progressive trend in heart rate should always be critically considered, an explanation found, and treatment adjusted appropriately. Heart rate is often the most sensitive indicator of response to treatment, especially infusion of fluid. The ECG rhythm should be carefully assessed.

Pulses

The character of pulses is helpful in assessing the state of the circulation and the presence or absence of specific pulses crucial to diagnosis of some congenital cardiac disorders. All major limb pulses should be palpated.

Colour and perfusion

This should be assessed in a semiquantitative way using the capillary refill test or peripheral temperature assessment. Look for differences in colour between the upper and lower body.

Level of consciousness

Low cardiac output causes first agitation then drowsiness and confusion.

Respiratory rate

A high respiratory rate is most commonly caused by respiratory disease, but is also an indirect indicator of cardiac output. It can be particularly useful when considered as a trend over a period of time.

Blood pressure

Normal blood pressure gives little indication on its own as to the cardiac output; a low blood pressure always indicates a serious problem.

Abdomen

The size of the liver is a useful indication of central venous pressure (CVP) in younger children and should be reassessed during therapy if CVP monitoring is not in place.

Monitoring

ECG and saturation monitoring are usually easy to arrange and should be the absolute minimum monitoring provided for intensive care transfers.

Non-invasive blood pressure is useful in the stable patient, but is a poor alternative to invasive monitoring and should only be used in unstable patients if there is no alternative.

Invasive pressure monitoring provides constant, accurate measurement as well as a waveform display. CVP monitoring is possible where central access has been gained. Interpretation of values can be made more difficult in transit by movement artefact.

End tidal CO_2, although generally considered a respiratory monitor, also reflects pulmonary blood flow.

Investigations

A number of investigations have specific relevance to the assessment of the cardiovascular system.

1. Blood gas. Provides information on the respiratory status, but is also useful in assessment of the cardiovascular system.

Acid–base balance of arterial blood indicates the adequacy of tissue oxygenation. The severity of acidosis gives an indirect assessment of the adequacy of cardiac output, as low cardiac output will lead to tissue hypoxia and metabolic acidosis.

2. Full blood count. Anaemia in any patient with shock or heart failure will exacerbate the problem and should be treated early in critically ill children.

3. The need to treat coagulopathy before transfer depends on the clinical situation. Premature infants are vulnerable to intracranial haemorrhage and should have a significant coagulopathy treated before or during transfer. Older children without evidence of haemorrhage may not require immediate treatment.

4. Blood electrolytes can have a significant effect on cardiac function, with blood calcium and potassium particularly important. Attempts should be made to correct abnormal values before transfer in unstable patients.

5. A chest radiograph can contribute to cardiac as well as respiratory status assessment. The heart size, pulmonary vascular markings, presence of effusions or pneumothorax, and the position of central venous lines should all be assessed.

Stabilisation

Vascular access

Stable venous access is a core requirement for safe transfer of unwell patients. As with all aspects of stabilisation, the transport environment makes it more likely that the patient will be unstable, more likely that access will fall out or fail, and much more difficult to replace if it does. It is often tempting to transfer a patient who has "just enough" venous access rather than to spend time gaining more. The high number of children who arrive at receiving hospitals *in extremis* because a drip failed, "tissued" or fell out during the transfer should be convincing evidence that the time is well spent.

Reliance on an ability to replace lines during transfer is unwise. In most situations it will be very difficult to achieve the same level of light and access to the patient as could be achieved in hospital. Even a stationary vehicle will be rocked by every passing car. In aircraft vibration makes performance of delicate procedures extremely difficult or impossible and there will be no option to "pull over" while the task is undertaken.

A good practice is to assume that at least one drip will fail during the transfer. This means that, at a minimum, there should be at least one more site of access available than is required at the time of departure. There should be enough access to continue all essential infusions as well as to give boluses of fluid or drugs. It can be seen that every unwell or ventilated patient will need two or more drips to meet this standard.

Peripheral venous access

The normal peripherally sited cannula can provide acceptable venous access for most patients. The skills required are generic and access can often be achieved quickly without much handling of the patient. Even narrow bore cannulas are short, allowing volume to be infused relatively quickly if sited in an adequate vein. Almost all drugs can be given into peripheral lines but may require dilution or special care.

There are some important disadvantages of reliance on peripheral lines. Each line has only one lumen so several may be required to achieve a safe transfer. In some patients it will be extremely difficult to gain access and, even if a line can be placed, it may not be possible to gain enough access for the transfer. Irritant substances cause phlebitis and it will be more difficult to detect that the line has tissued during the transfer than in normal circumstances.

Central venous access

Central access has a number of advantages over peripheral lines. Multiple lumens may be placed at one time, lines do not tissue in the short term, fixation of the line is often easier, irritant and vasoactive drugs may be given at high concentration, and venous pressure may be monitored if required.

Access in the newborn is often achieved via the umbilical vein. This is a generic skill and can usually be achieved quickly even in extremely premature infants. Securing the line can be difficult and care should be taken to avoid traction on the line.

After the newborn period access to the central veins must be by percutaneous insertion. This is slower and more difficult than umbilical vein cannulation, especially in small infants. There is a higher risk of immediate side effects as a needle must be passed blindly into the target vein. Internal jugular, subclavian or femoral veins may be used.

The advantages of having central access indicate obtaining it at a low threshold when preparing unwell patients for transport. Clinicians should, however, recognise that alternative strategies are usually available if they do not have sufficient experience of percutaneous techniques to attempt this safely.

Inotropes

Inotropes are a useful group of drugs that all increase either the cardiac output or the blood pressure.

In situations where cardiac dysfunction is likely to be present inotropes should be used early. This includes extremely premature infants for whom the importance of establishing an adequate and stable blood pressure has been mentioned. In the presence of cardiac failure repeated boluses of fluid can cause increasing cardiac dilatation and deterioration of the patient's condition. Particularly in infants with a history that is compatible with cardiac disease, clinicians should remain alert to deterioration associated with fluid administration and modify their treatment appropriately.

The effects of the most commonly used inotropes are summarised in Table 9.4.

Intravenous fluids and blood products

Increasing the amount and pressure of fluid returning to the heart is usually the quickest and simplest way to increase cardiac output. The best fluid to administer depends on what, if any, fluid has been lost.

In the short term 0·9% saline is an effective and available fluid with which to increase the circulating volume of blood. Many centres use plasma or albumin solutions in the hope that these will remain inside the circulation for longer than saline, but there is little evidence that this is true.

Use of dextrose or hypotonic saline (less than 0·9%) to increase circulating volume is disastrous as the fluid is immediately lost from the circulation and contributes only to the formation of oedema and electrolyte disturbance.

The amount of fluid administered must be tailored to the clinical situation. During initial

Table 9.4 Effects of most commonly used inotropes

Drug	Cardiac output	Vascular resistance	Effect
Dopamine	↑	↑ ↑↑ (high dose)	Increases cardiac output and blood pressure
Dobutamine	↑	—	Increases cardiac output but variable effect on blood pressure
Epinephrine (adrenaline)	↑	↑ ↑↑↑ (high dose)	Increases cardiac output and blood pressure
Norepinephrine (noradrenaline)	—	↑↑↑	Increases blood pressure but little direct effect on cardiac output
Milrinone	↑	↓	Increases cardiac output but may decrease blood pressure

resuscitation seriously shocked or hypotensive patients who do not have obvious cardiac disease should receive an initial bolus of 20 ml/kg. Monitored patients should receive smaller volumes and the patient's response noted. This can be given as quickly or as frequently as required as long as it is tailored to the patient's response. The need for large volumes of fluid should prompt consideration of inotrope use or the possibility of haemorrhage.

Children with cardiac disease may deteriorate rapidly during fluid administration. Small volumes should be used when cardiac disease is a possible diagnosis and inotropes introduced at an early stage.

A slow infusion of maintenance fluids may be used to maintain blood glucose and electrolyte levels. Premature and newborn infants will require a constant glucose infusion. This may not be necessary in older children during short distance transfers.

Arrhythmias

In paediatric intensive care units infants who have had recent cardiac surgery are the group most likely to suffer cardiac rhythm abnormalities. Luckily, this group tends not to require interhospital transfer. Other groups who are prone to arrhythmias include children: who have had cardiac surgery in the past; with a congenital predisposition to arrhythmias (e.g. supraventricular tachycardia and long QT syndrome); who have ingested toxic levels of drugs (e.g. tricyclic antidepressants); and those who have myocarditis or a cardiomyopathy.

Ways of preventing arrhythmia

- Effectively treat hypoxia and hypercarbia
- Detect and treat hypo- and hyperkalaemia
- Detect and treat hypo- and hypercalcaemia
- Alkalinisation of child who has taken tricyclics
- Ensure continuance of antidysrhythmic medication
- Ensure adequate coronary blood flow and diastolic BP and observe ST segments.

CLINICAL APPROACH
If a child has an arrhythmia, examine:
- the child
then
- the child's ECG

Approach to the ECG
Always feel a pulse before looking at the ECG

Question	Answer
1. Can you see P waves regularly associated with normal QRS complex? Is heart rate < 200?	Yes Sinus rhythm (fast or slow)
2. Is the heart rate > 220 (relatively fixed P waves may or may not be visible)? Normal narrow QRS complex?	Yes SVT
3. Broad complex tachycardia Rate almost constant (between 120 and 250/min) Sustained > 3 beats	Yes VT
4. Irregular bizarre complexes of fine or coarse nature (ensure adequate gain on monitor)	Yes VF

Staff preparing to transfer a patient who has had or is at risk of having an arrhythmia should discuss treatment with a paediatric cardiologist or intensivist. All staff need to be able to recognise the most common and arrest arrhythmias and should be able to safely use a defibrillator. An appropriate defibrillator needs to be immediately available throughout the transfer. Unstable patients should have defibrillation pads attached to avoid use of paddles where this is possible.

Many teams do not carry their own defibrillator on transfers and depend on equipment carried by the ambulance service. In this situation it is important to check that the defibrillator available is appropriate for the patient. Some ambulance services use semiautomatic defibrillators that cannot be adjusted for use in children.

How the team will react in the event of the patient having an arrhythmia should be discussed before leaving. It is often better for the ambulance crew to operate ambulance equipment guided by transfer team staff than to attempt to use unfamiliar equipment in an emergency.

Congenital cardiac disease

Children with congenital cardiac disease represent a high proportion of patients managed in many paediatric intensive care units. Initial presentation, however, is often to neonatal, accident and emergency or general paediatric departments. Transfer to a cardiology or cardiac intensive care unit will be required.

Cardiac malformations that present in the newborn period usually do so because they cause either obstruction of blood flow to the lungs or obstruction of blood flow to the systemic circulation (the rest of the body).

Narrowing or blockage of the pulmonary artery or valve or failure of the right ventricle to form will result in blood flowing from the aorta to the pulmonary artery through the ductus arteriosus. This allows the infant to survive after birth. Oxygen saturations will be lower than normal as there is mixing of oxygenated and deoxygenated blood, but the infant may appear well and be discharged from the maternity unit. When the ductus starts to close the infant will quickly become hypoxic as blood flow to the lungs decreases. This will cause deep cyanosis followed by collapse.

Narrowing or obstruction of the aorta, or failure of the left ventricle to form, results in blood flowing from the pulmonary artery to the aorta through the ductus. Again, oxygen saturations will be low as there is mixing of oxygenated and deoxygenated blood but the infant may appear generally well. As the ductus closes blood flow into the aorta will decrease and the infant will become shocked. The oxygen saturation may actually increase at this stage as most of the cardiac output is being directed to the lungs.

Reopening the duct is essential in both these groups of patients. This is done with an infusion of prostaglandin E2 (Prostin). A normal starting dose of Prostin is 10 nanograms (0·01 micrograms) per kilogram per minute. This may be increased if there is no initial response and can usually be decreased in stable patients for use over longer periods.

Patients diagnosed as having a potentially duct dependent circulation (Box 9.1) while still well should be started on Prostin to prevent duct closure.

- Overall about 80% of infants respond.
- The response is usually evident within 15 minutes.
- If in doubt start the infusion.
- Infants with total anomalous pulmonary venous drainage (TAPVD) may get worse in which case stop the infusion.

Box 9.1   Examples of ductus dependent lesions

Decreased pulmonary flow:
  Tricuspid atresia
  Pulmonary atresia
  Critical pulmonary stenosis
  Transposition of great arteries

Decreased systemic flow:
  Hypoplastic left heart
  Coarctation of aorta
  Critical aortic valve stenosis
  Interrupted aortic arch

One of the important side effects of Prostin is its tendency to cause apnoea and this should be taken into consideration when planning transfer of the patient. The risk of apnoea is usually transient and most commonly associated with use of higher doses (doses of more than 0·01 micrograms/kg/min (10 nanograms/kg/min)). Elective intubation and ventilation should be considered for stable infants who are to be transferred immediately after starting Prostin therapy. Infants who have not suffered apnoea after several hours of Prostin infusion are unlikely to do so and ventilation is not generally necessary. Other side effects of Prostin infusion are:

- Vasodilatation
- Hypotension (mild)
- Jitteriness
- Fever.

If jitteriness or fever occur consider halving the infusion rate.

Practicalities of prostaglandin infusion

Prostaglandin E2 (Prostin E2, dinoprostone) is administered intravenously in a starting dose of 0·003–0·01 micrograms/kg/min (3–10 nanograms/kg/min).

Dilution

1. Take ampoule of PGE_2 (1 mg/ml) and draw up 1 ml (1 mg) into a syringe—do not remove the needle.
2. Inject 1 ml (1 mg) of PGE_2 from the syringe into a 500 ml bag of 5% dextrose or 0·9% saline
3. Mix well. This solution now contains 2 micrograms/ml of PGE_2.
4. Start IV infusion at the rate of 0·3 ml/kg/h. This is 0·01 micrograms/kg/min (10 nanograms/kg/min). Round off the infusion rate to the nearest 0·1 ml; for example, for a 3·5 kg infant the initial estimated infusion rate is 0·3 ml × 3·5 = 1·05 ml/h—infuse at 1·0 ml/h.

Increase the rate of infusion in multiples of 0·1 ml/kg/h to a maximum of 0·6 ml/kg/h (0·02 micrograms/kg/min) depending upon the clinical response. Doses above this may be needed, particularly in the shocked patient, but advice should be sought from a paediatric cardiologist. Once a sustained clinical improvement is attained (a rise in Pao_2 or improvement in heart failure), the dose should be reduced in similar steps to below 0·01 micrograms/kg/min.

Do not use the intra-arterial route, except in an emergency—although it is equally effective, side effects are common.

Particular congenital heart lesions (Table 9.5)

The most common cardiac malformations are defects in the septum between the ventricles or atria. The most severe have both atrial and ventricular defects and may be associated with heart valve abnormalities.

These conditions rarely present at birth, although they may be detected on routine examination. As pulmonary vascular resistance drops over the first weeks of life pulmonary blood flow increases and the patient will present with signs of heart failure. The oxygen saturations will be normal until pulmonary oedema causes respiratory hypoxia. It is unusual for this group of patients to collapse suddenly unless they develop an intercurrent illness, such as bronchiolitis, which is exacerbated by their underlying cardiac condition.

The ductus arteriosus may fail to close in some children. This allows blood flow from the aorta to the pulmonary artery, causing increased pulmonary blood flow and occasionally heart failure. This is particularly common in premature infants in whom it can exacerbate lung disease and may prevent weaning from ventilation. Patients may require transfer to a cardiac unit for ligation of the ductus.

Hypoplastic left heart

Infants usually present with severe ventricular failure and cyanosis.

If active treatment is planned, treatment should include:

- Ventilation:
    - Ketamine and suxamethonium induction
    - Target $Paco_2$ 5 kPa
    - Target Sao_2 75%
    - Adequate sedation with opiate
- Prostaglandin in infants less than 14 days old
- Inotrope (usually epinephrine (adrenaline))
- Furosemide (frusemide) 1 mg/kg IV.

Tetralogy of Fallot—hypercyanotic spells

As the right ventricular outflow tract (RVOT) hypertrophies, a dynamic RVOT obstruction may develop, presenting as episodic severe cyanosis—hypercyanotic spells.

Treatment aims to:

- Reduce RVOT obstruction
- Increase systemic vascular resistance.

Systemic vascular resistance is increased by initially encouraging the knee–chest position, then

Table 9.5 Common cyanotic conditions

Transposition of great arteries	Tetralogy of Fallot	Pulmonary atresia or tricuspid atresia	Anomalous pulmonary venous drainage
History of cyanosis Early onset implies no or restrictive VSD Late onset usually with congestive failure (and VSD)	History May be pink until infundibulum hypertrophies SPELLS may occur Cyanosis from birth implies severe RVOT obstruction	History Onset at birth usually as ductus closes Later onset if VSD with evidence of ventricular failure	History Very variable onset Early onset implies all pulmonary venous drainage anomalous + probably restricted usually associated with ventricular failure Later onset with ventricular failure
Examination Pulse often normal Hyperdynamic apex Often little to find	Examination Normal pulse Right ventricular heave Pulmonary ejection murmur Single P2	Examination Severe cyanosis PA = single P2 TA = pansystolic murmur Praecordium hyperdynamic	Examination Cyanosis with ventricular failure Often little else to find
ECG Normal	ECG Axis +90–180° Right ventricular hypertrophy	ECG PA = QRS 0–90° P pulmonale TA = QRS −90–+90 P pulmonale	ECG Right ventricular hypertrophy P pulmonale
CXR Cardiomegaly—increased pulmonary flow	CXR Normal heart size, upturned apex Empty pulmonary bay Reduced pulmonary flow (20% right aortic arch)	CXR Decreased pulmonary flow	CXR Right ventricle + pulmonary artery prominent Increased pulmonary flow

VSD = ventricular septal defect, RVOT = right ventricular outflow tract, PA = pulmonary atresia, TA = tricuspid atresia.

consideration of the following drugs, often used sequentially until effective:

1. Morphine 10 micrograms/kg IV or 25 micrograms/kg IM
2. Sodium bicarbonate 1 mmol/kg IV initially
3. Infuse 10 ml/kg colloid or crystalloid
4. Esmolol 0·25 mg/kg over 1 minute then 50 micrograms/kg/min. If ineffective by 5 minutes repeat with 0·5 mg/kg and up to 250 micrograms/kg/min
5. Phenylephrine 2–10 micrograms/kg stat, then 1–5 micrograms/kg/min.

Be prepared to ventilate.

Conditions palliated with a shunt that has blocked

The following conditions may be palliated by shunting between systemic and pulmonary circulations:

- Tetralogy of Fallot
- Pulmonary atresia
- Tricuspid atresia.

Blockage of the shunt is usually characterised by cyanosis:

- Heart failure
- Extreme cyanosis
- Absence of shunt murmur.

It is important to reach a cardiac centre quickly having initiated:

- Ventilation
- Inotropic support (usually epinephrine (adrenaline))
- Diuretic.

Transposition of the great arteries

Although there is no actual obstruction in transposition, the circulation is dependent on both the ductus arteriosus and the foramen ovale to allow blood from the pulmonary and systemic circulations to mix. In addition to starting a Prostin infusion it is often necessary to enlarge the foramen ovale. A "septostomy" is performed by a cardiologist using a device threaded into a large vein under echocardiogram guidance. This is rarely possible outside a paediatric cardiology centre so transfer should not be excessively delayed. It will occasionally not be possible to fully stabilise the patient before transfer.

Summary
In unwell infants and children who require interhospital transfer, stabilisation of the circulation is essential to ensure the transfer is safe and to avoid the long term consequences of instability.
Stabilisation should be approached as it is within the intensive care unit and based on a detailed history, careful review of information, and clinical examination of the patient.
Sufficient monitoring and vascular access must be established before transfer to continue all aspects of intensive care and to compensate for the difficulties associated with the transport environment. Transferring staff should have a low threshold for establishing central venous access and using inotrope infusions.
Children with congenital cardiac disease require specialist care and are therefore often transferred between hospitals.
The use of Prostin to open the ductus arteriosus is central to the stabilisation of infants with congenital cardiac disease presenting in the newborn period.

10 Trauma

Introduction

In the UK trauma is the commonest cause of death in children over the age of one. However, as the overall incidence of severe injury is relatively small, most clinicians dealing with these children on an infrequent basis will transfer them to major centres for definitive care. The Trauma Audit and Research Network (TARN) recorded that between 1991 and the end of 2001 there were 20 492 children (aged less than 16) requiring some form of transfer to another centre in the 103 hospitals contributing to TARN. Of these, 31% had Injury Severity Scores exceeding 9, suggestive of severe injury.

When considering transfer it is essential that:

- All injuries which may compromise safe transfer are recognised. Operative intervention may be required to stabilise the patient prior to transfer
- The benefits of transferring the patient to the receiving hospital significantly outweigh the risks of the transfer itself
- The optimal time for transfer is identified and the transport team has all the capabilities required to carry it out safely.

Objectives

To understand:

- The mechanics and resulting patterns of injury in infants and children
- Clinical assessment of the child prior to transfer, using the system of a primary and secondary survey, with particular emphasis on the need to:
  exclude life or limb threatening pathology
  recognise the potential for acute decompensation in certain body regions
- A review of important injuries within individual body regions of particular relevance for transfer
- Practical procedures relevant to transferring the injured child
- Analgesia issues in the trauma patient
- Documentation issues prior to transfer
- Pitfalls in transferring the injured child.

The mechanics and resulting injury patterns

Major traumatic injury produces markedly different physiological and physical effects on children as compared to adults.

Children are often prone to injuries as a result of road traffic accidents (RTAs) and falls. Most commonly, a child is involved in an accident with a vehicle as a pedestrian or cyclist, rather than as a car occupant. The inquisitive nature of small children, and their lack of appreciation of danger, also predisposes them to injuries from falls. Multisystem injury may be the result, and it is prudent to base the initial assessment on this assumption until proven otherwise.

Three factors influencing the resulting injury patterns are discussed below.

Size

Due to the smaller body mass and relative size of children, the patterns of injury are different to those of an adult for the following reasons.

- Collision with a vehicle imparts a greater force per unit body area.
- Multiple organs are in close proximity to one another.
- The child's body has less fat, muscle and elastic connective tissue to absorb the traumatic forces.

For example, a child knocked down by a car is at significant risk of pelvic and abdominal injuries as opposed to lower limb fractures in an adult; a child has a disproportionately large head and is at greater risk of a severe head injury after a fall.

Surface area

The ratio of a child's body surface area to volume is highest at birth and diminishes as the child reaches adolescence. As a result, hypothermia may develop rapidly and complicate the management of the traumatised child. Therefore:

- Exposure of the injured child must be kept to a minimum
- Use warmed blankets and fluids
- Children with burns can very rapidly become hypothermic, especially if wet clothes and dressings are applied.

Skeleton

The child's skeleton is incompletely calcified and is more pliable. As a result, internal organ damage may occur without overlying bony injury.

- Rib fractures are uncommon but pulmonary contusion is frequent.
- There is little protection to the liver, spleen and kidneys from the overlying ribs.
- Rib and pelvic fractures are rare, but their presence implies massive traumatic forces that will have been transmitted to the underlying thoracic and abdominal contents.

Clinical assessment

The emergency management of the critically injured child relies on the assessment and treatment of hypoxia and shock, as well as on the identification of injuries and early access to definitive care in a timely fashion. This approach is structured into a primary and secondary survey as set out by the Advanced Trauma Life Support (ATLS) course.

Prior to transfer, a primary and secondary review must be performed and the findings documented. This reassessment effectively constitutes a tertiary survey, and is specifically targeted at identifying any potential or actual life threatening emergencies. These may have developed, or have been overlooked, during the initial assessment and resuscitation.

Failure to perform a tertiary survey will compromise the quality of a stable transfer. This survey, and the appropriate management of any problems identified, should occur in a timely fashion, as the transfer itself may be for urgent definitive treatment of injuries. The tertiary transport survey should end with a clear management plan, outlining the needs both of the patient and the transfer team.

Primary review

The primary review is divided into five parts. It is used as a rapid and logical method to identify any immediate or impending life-threatening pathology. The same system is regularly used to re-evaluate the patient during the transfer itself.

A. Airway and cervical spine control

Assessment of the airway is critical to a safe transfer. Trauma patients will fall into two broad categories.

- The alert, conscious patient will have a clear airway and no further interventions will be necessary apart from oxygen therapy.

- The patient with a compromised airway, or one where there is potential for compromise. Prior to transfer, the patient must be anaesthetised and the airway secured by endotracheal intubation.

Common indications for securing the airway include:

- The need to protect the lower airway from aspiration of blood or vomit. Always assume the trauma patient to have a full stomach with delayed gastric emptying
- Impending or potential airway compromise; for example, following facial burns or inhalational injury, facial trauma, or epileptic seizures
- Closed head injury with potential for neurological deterioration
- Inability to maintain adequate oxygenation and gas exchange
- High spinal cord injuries.

Once the child is intubated and sedated, frequent re-evaluation of the airway is vital.

Monitor physiological parameters and check oxygen supply, ventilator settings, circuit and connections regularly. Be aware of dislodgement (main bronchus or oesophagus) or blockage of the endotracheal tube. Visualise chest expansion and check for pneumothorax.

Cervical spine immobilisation must be maintained at all times in any patient with a potentially severe injury. Clearance of the child's spine may occur only after both clinical and radiological assessment by an experienced clinician.

Learning points
Any doubt about an airway prior to transfer should suggest the need to secure it by endotracheal intubation.
In the anaesthetised child, ensure that the endotracheal tube is secured by at least two methods.
An orogastric or nasogastric tube should be inserted prior to transfer in all anaesthetised children.

B. Breathing

Careful assessment is essential to identify signs of respiratory distress compromising ventilatory function. Examination of the chest must be linked with a review of changes in respiratory rate, oxygen saturation, and arterial blood gas analysis. Chest pathology in the injured child is easily missed. Important causes include tension pneumothorax; simple pneumothorax; haemo-thorax; splinting of the diaphragm due to gastric dilatation; pulmonary contusion or even a flail chest.

> *Learning points*
> Tension pneumothorax may manifest at any time, especially after the child has been anaesthetised and endotracheally intubated. Consider it in all cases where acute compromise occurs.
> Beware of pulmonary contusion. Due to the compliance of the chest wall, there may be few signs of severe chest trauma until manifest as hypoxia and respiratory distress.

C. Circulation

All patients must be cardiovascularly stable prior to transfer. Initial assessment will have been based upon the pulse rate and volume, capillary refill, conscious state, and respiratory rate. Blood pressure is a poor sign of cardiovascular compromise.

It is essential to examine the charts and review the impact of fluids given to the patient. If more than 40 ml/kg of fluid has been given to resuscitate the child, a possible source for haemorrhage must be identified. Review possible causes of hidden cavity blood loss and ensure that an experienced surgeon has assessed the patient prior to transfer.

> *Learning points*
> Blood loss may be obvious (scalp laceration, fractured long bones) or occult (into the chest, abdomen, retroperitoneum, or pelvis). The patient may require operative intervention to control the haemorrhage prior to transfer.
> In rare circumstances, once hypovolaemia has been excluded, there may be other causes for shock (cardiogenic from myocardial contusion or neurogenic from spinal cord injury).
> It is essential to have all vascular lines well secured prior to transfer.

D. Disability assessment

A review of the patient's neurological state is essential prior to transfer. The assessment of the Glasgow Coma Score at this stage is difficult as most patients with significant head injuries will have been anaesthetised and given paralysing agents. It is important, however, to elicit and document the pupillary responses.

E. Exposure and environment control

Measures to minimise heat loss should be instituted prior to, and especially during, the transfer. A core temperature must be documented and monitored during transfer.

Secondary review

The secondary review allows the transport team to:

- Familiarise themselves with the injuries that have been identified thus far
- Identify other injuries that may influence the transfer of the patient.

The review should be a thorough head to toe examination. It is best carried out with the team that was initially taking care of the patient. This review may identify the need for further urgent investigations or treatment prior to transfer. However, it should also be done in a timely fashion and take into account the urgency of the situation.

A clear management plan should be formulated and documented at this stage. Details of specific personnel involved in the referring and receiving hospital as well as the exact destination must also be recorded.

The next section concentrates on important injuries within each of the individual body regions.

Head injury

Children with head injuries constitute the largest single group of transfers due to trauma. Head injuries account for 15% of all deaths in the 1–15 year age group. This is most commonly due to collisions with vehicles and to falls. In infancy, the most common cause is child abuse. The overall outcome in children suffering a severe head injury is better than in adults.

Transfer may be indicated for specialised intensive care facilities, intracranial pressure (ICP) monitoring, or for neurosurgery.

Intracranial pressure

Children tend to have fewer focal mass lesions than adults, but raised ICP due to cerebral oedema is more common.

Normal ICP in the resting state is 10 mmHg. In trauma, both cerebral oedema and intracranial haematoma (ICH) can cause raised ICP, the presence of which not only indicates intracranial pathology, but also exacerbates it in a vicious cycle.

Monro–Kellie doctrine

This is a simple concept in which the cranial cavity can be considered as a fixed-volume box, so that the total volume of intracranial contents must remain constant.

If cerebral oedema or ICH occurs, compensatory mechanisms maintain normal ICP by squeezing an equal volume of CSF and venous blood out of the cranial cavity.

Once these mechanisms are exhausted, decompensation occurs and ICP rises in an exponential manner until the stage at which cerebral herniation occurs.

In children this pathophysiological mechanism applies only after fusion of the cranial sutures (between 12 and 18 months).

Whilst the sutures are open:

- There is greater allowance for intracranial volume expansion
- Intracranial haemorrhage and/or oedema may occur before neurological symptoms or signs develop
- An infant with a bulging fontanelle or suture diastasis should be treated as having a severe head injury.

Raised ICP causes an increased pressure gradient for the inflow of arterial blood and therefore a fall in cerebral perfusion pressure (CPP).

Cerebral perfusion pressure

Both normal and injured brain tissue must remain adequately perfused to prevent irreversible damage and to preserve function.

CPP = mean arterial blood pressure − ICP

Blood pressure must be maintained in the head injured patient, particularly in the presence of:

- Raised ICP
- Multiple injuries.

Management priorities

Children are particularly susceptible to the effects of secondary brain injury. The first priority must be to prevent this by ensuring adequate cerebral perfusion with well oxygenated blood.

- Assessment and stabilisation of the airway, breathing and circulation is mandatory.
- The airway must be protected with an appropriately sized endotracheal tube and the child ventilated after administration of muscle relaxants and sedation.
- Correction of hypovolaemia and maintenance of adequate blood pressure are paramount.
- Early liaison with the regional paediatric neurosurgical centre is vital.
- Raised ICP may be apparent clinically or radiologically; follow neurosurgical advice regarding treatment.

Focal mass lesions

A CT head scan is required to visualise focal mass lesions, but these occur less frequently in children.

Prevention of secondary brain injury

- Hypoxia. Ensure adequate oxygenation at all times.
- Hyper- or hypocapnia. Maintain Pa_{CO_2} at the lower range of normal (4·0 kPa) to prevent cerebral vasodilatation. Note that hypocapnia will cause marked vasoconstriction and impair cerebral perfusion.
- Hypovolaemia. Monitor physiological parameters and capillary refill. Assess response to fluids and urinary output. Exclude ongoing blood loss. Consider invasive monitoring of arterial pressure and central venous pressure.
- Seizures. Control early with lorazepam and phenytoin. Suspect seizure activity in the paralysed patient if there is a sharp increase in heart rate and blood pressure with dilatation of the pupils.
- Hypoglycaemia.
- Anaemia.

Temporary measures to counteract raised ICP

- Nurse in the 30° head up position.
- Infusion of IV mannitol (0·5–1·0 g/kg) after neurosurgical advice.
- Maintain the Pa_{CO_2} at the lower range of normal; use of the end tidal CO_2 (ET_{CO_2}) monitor will help to prevent hyperventilation.

Investigations prior to transfer

Blood tests

Review the results of blood tests and correct abnormalities. Review the indications for cross-matched blood and ensure that it is available for transfer.

Radiographs

Review the *x* ray films of the cervical spine, chest, and pelvis, as well as those indicated during the secondary survey. Ensure that a decision is made as to whether the entire spinal column has been cleared, otherwise immobilisation must continue.

CT scans

Consult local guidelines on the indications for a CT head scan which should be performed early. The neurosurgical centre must be contacted with the clinical details and results of the scan. Often, the CT images can be transmitted simultaneously and delays to transfer minimised. If CT scanning is unavailable then the child should be transferred after neurosurgical consultation on the phone.

Learning points
A decrease in the level of consciousness may indicate decreased cerebral perfusion or be due to direct cerebral injury.
An altered level of consciousness indicates a need to re-evaluate the patient's oxygenation, ventilation and perfusion status.
If hypoxia and hypovolaemia are excluded, changes in the level of consciousness should be considered to be of a traumatic CNS origin until proven otherwise.

Chest injury

Ten per cent of all injuries from trauma involve the chest. Always consider thoracic injury in children with multiple injuries.

Children have a very pliable chest wall, and in trauma significant kinetic energy transfer may occur without external signs of injury. As a result rib fracture is rare but pulmonary contusion is common.

Pulmonary contusion

- Pulmonary contusion may not become apparent either clinically or radiologically until after the first few hours.
- The injury is the result of rupture of pulmonary capillaries and alveolar haemorrhage.
- The child will become progressively more hypoxic, requiring higher concentrations of Fio_2.
- Gas exchange and pulmonary mechanics may significantly deteriorate unless recognised and anticipated early.
- Thoracic CT is a sensitive imaging modality for pulmonary contusion, especially when the initial chest radiograph is non-diagnostic.

If the child is shocked the following life threatening injuries must be excluded.

- Tension pneumothorax. Air accumulates in the pleural space, pushing the mediastinum across the chest and compromising venous return to the heart.
- Massive haemothorax. A significant proportion of the child's blood volume accumulates in the pleural space from parenchymal, pulmonary and chest wall damage.
- Rare injuries include flail chest, cardiac tamponade, open pneumothorax, disruption of the major airway and great vessels, and diaphragmatic rupture.

Management priorities

- Recognise the signs of increased work of breathing and hypoxia.
- Provide high concentrations of oxygen and monitor closely.
- Have a low threshold for intubation and positive pressure ventilation (IPPV).
- Establish clear indications for an intercostal chest drain.
- Be aware of clinically important complications of chest drains.
- If sudden deterioration occurs always consider tension pneumothorax.

The risk of a tension pneumothorax is increased in the following circumstances.

- Occlusion of a chest drain, for example kinked or clamped.
- Misplacement or inadvertent removal of a chest drain.
- The presence of rib fractures and IPPV.
- An undrained pneumothorax and IPPV.

> *Learning points*
> Complications of IPPV:
>   Failure to correct hypovolaemia prior to anaesthesia and IPPV may result in profound hypotension.
>   Tension pneumothorax may develop after IPPV in thoracic trauma.
> Complications of chest drains:
>   Assign a member of the transport team to be responsible for the chest drain during movement of the child, to minimise the risks of occlusion or withdrawal.

Abdominal injury

The abdomen presents a diagnostic challenge in the traumatised child; occult haemorrhage needs to be excluded before considering transfer.

If haemodynamic stability has not been achieved after 40 ml/kg fluid resuscitation, then thoracic, abdominal or pelvic haemorrhage is likely.

A senior and experienced surgeon must be involved early if abdominal trauma has occurred, especially if the child has been shocked.

A combination of factors makes the abdominal contents of the child very susceptible to injury.

- The abdominal muscles are thin and offer little protection.
- The liver and spleen are lower and more anterior due to a relatively flat diaphragm.
- The compliant lower chest wall offers little protection to the underlying organs.
- The full bladder is intra-abdominal rather than pelvic.

Patterns of injury

- Deceleration injuries. Cause differential movement between fixed and mobile organs; for example, falls from a height and RTAs may cause liver and spleen lacerations and disruption.
- Shearing forces. Cause a crushing-type injury when a restraint device such as a seat-belt (lap-belt or shoulder harness) is incorrectly worn, causing solid organ disruption and mesenteric injuries.
- Compression or crushing injury. Causes contusion and rupture of solid and hollow organs; for example, a direct blow from a punch or bicycle handlebars may cause duodenal or pancreatic contusion, a punch to the full bladder may cause rupture.

- Straddling injuries. Cause perineal and urethral injury, for example from a fall or bicycle accident.

Management priorities

The potential for abdominal trauma must be continually reassessed, if not immediately apparent during the primary and secondary surveys.

- Prior to considering transfer, intra-abdominal injury must be confidently excluded.
- Any child with blunt traumatic injuries adjacent to the abdomen must be considered to have an intra-abdominal injury until it is excluded.
- If there is any uncertainty, particularly in children with head or spinal injuries, then the senior surgeon must decide whether abdominal ultrasound, CT scanning or laparotomy is indicated.
- If haemoperitoneum is identified then non-operative management is not an option for the child being transferred.

Pelvic fractures

Pelvic fractures are relatively uncommon in children but when they occur can cause life threatening haemorrhage.

Senior orthopaedic staff must be involved early if pelvic fracture is identified. The pelvis may need emergency stabilisation to control haemorrhage (external fixation or a pneumatic anti-shock garment).

Spinal injury

Spinal injury is relatively rare in children. This relates partly to the anatomical differences. There is greater laxity in the interspinous ligaments and joint capsules. In addition the vertebral bodies are wedged anteriorly and therefore tend to slide forwards with flexion. It is essential, however, to maintain a high index of suspicion based upon the mechanism of injury.

Assessment is particularly difficult if the child is unconscious, frightened, or in pain. Immobilisation techniques are outlined below under "Practical procedures".

Spinal injury is almost always located in the cervical region in children. This relates to the relatively large head and the flexibility of the cervical spine in the younger child. Thoracolumbar injuries, when they occur, are usually in children with multiple injuries.

Plain radiology is helpful in detecting pathology but can be compromised by:

- Difficulties in interpreting plain *x* ray films due to ossification centres, physeal lines, and pseudosubluxation of C2 on C3, and C3 on C4
- The presence of spinal cord injury without radiological abnormality (SCIWORA). Although this is a rare phenomenon, this probably relates to the infrequency of spinal cord injury itself in children. The incidence in one series is reported to be 55% of patients with confirmed spinal cord injury.

It is important to re-evaluate the clinical signs of spinal cord injury prior to transfer to a specialist centre and clearly document these findings.

High dose steroids may be indicated within the first eight hours of spinal cord injury. Discuss the case with the specialist centre and take advice. Also seek advice on the need to catheterise the child and the type of catheter to use.

Consider spinal cord injury and neurogenic shock in a patient with hypotension and/or a relative bradycardia, where hypovolaemia has been excluded. This is due to loss of vasomotor tone caused by disruption of the descending sympathetic pathways in the spinal cord. Judicious use of fluid therapy and possibly vasopressors are required. Seek specialist advice.

Transfer with spinal immobilisation can present management difficulties. Some ambulance services use ordinary scoop stretchers in preference to the spinal board. An alternative is the vacuum mattress which is discussed further below. The problems with the spinal board include: inadequate support and immobilisation, especially with small children; increased risk of pressure sores; and pain and discomfort in the conscious child. Advanced planning is recommended so that the child is securely immobilised to prevent any significant movement.

> *Learning points*
> The golden rule is to continue spinal immobilisation until clinical examination and relevant investigations by experienced personnel can exclude injury.

Extremity trauma

Limb injuries are common reasons for admitting children to hospital following trauma. The initial resuscitation and secondary review will identify the three main groups of patients.

1. Those with potential life threatening consequences, for example multiple limb fractures, crush injuries, traumatic amputation.

   a. Follow the ABCs. Prevent further haemorrhage with pressure dressings and traction splints (see below).
   b. Give fluids to achieve cardiovascular stability. Ensure blood is given early.
   c. Give broad spectrum antibiotics and check tetanus status.
   d. Store an amputated limb in the appropriate medium (wrap in moist dressings, place in a sealed plastic bag, and surround the bag with crushed ice and water).

2. Injuries leading to progressive limb or joint threatening conditions, for example acute compartment syndrome, vascular compromise due to joint disruption, or vascular injury itself due to a penetrating cause.

   a. Positively look for, and exclude, acute compartment syndrome. This occurs due to a rise in pressure in any fascial compartment within the body. The commonest and most important signs are acute pain on passively stretching the muscles involved and swelling of the affected limb. The first may be negated if the child is unconscious. Sensory disturbance in the distribution of the nerves running through the affected compartment may be present but can be difficult to elicit and is a poor sign. If in doubt, discuss the case with a senior orthopaedic surgeon. This is a true orthopaedic emergency.
   b. A dislocated joint—commonly the elbow or ankle—is best relocated prior to the transfer. This may be performed under sedation or general anaesthetic, depending upon the age of the patient.
   c. Acute vascular disruption. Absent or weak distal pulses on clinical examination or Doppler ultrasound suggest arterial injury. Angiography is required to identify pathology.

The severity of these injuries themselves may be a reason for transferring the patient, or they may be of secondary importance to other life threatening pathology.

3. Isolated limb fractures that may be open (compound) or closed.

   a. These may cause difficulties in intravenous or intraosseous access. Insertion of a femoral line or venous cutdown are alternatives in these circumstances.

   b. Remember that blood loss is proportionately greater into a fractured long bone or a pelvic fracture than in an adult.

   c. Ensure appropriate pain control for transfer. Limb splintage is discussed below.

> *Learning points*
> Compartment syndrome may be difficult to diagnose in unconscious or anaesthetised patients.
> Excessive, abnormal movement of broken limbs may compromise vessels, exacerbate haemorrhage, and cause pain.
> Ensure that all major fractures are appropriately splinted and that compound injuries are covered with appropriate saline-soaked or Betadine dressings.

Burns

Children suffering burns constitute a significant proportion of children requiring transportation to specialised centres. All staff should be aware of the transfer criteria of their local burns centre. The resuscitation priorities are the same as described above. A number of additional points require emphasis.

The primary review

It is most important to decide if the child has any signs that might suggest the potential for airway compromise. Patients at risk include those with facial burns or singed eyebrows, inhalational steam burns, and those with carbonaceous sputum. In such circumstances, it is essential to secure the airway by endotracheal intubation prior to transfer.

Consider other causes for respiratory distress. These may be due to mechanical causes as a result of circumferential burns or chest pathology from a fall.

It is essential to measure carboxyhaemoglobin, to exclude carbon monoxide poisoning, if there is any suggestion of smoke inhalation from entrapment in a confined space. Cellular hypoxia may also be a result of cyanide poisoning.

Circulatory compromise should be treated with a fluid bolus of 20 ml/kg of body weight and the response assessed.

Search for any signs of coexisting trauma if there is any suggestion of a fall (for example, from a house fire). Spinal immobilisation is then also necessary, as well as the exclusion of other life threatening pathology.

Assessment of the burn size

Clear documentation must identify the exact time and extent of the burn, as well as the fluids given since the time of injury.

The total body surface area (BSA) burnt in children is best calculated using the Lund and Browder charts (Fig. 10.1, Table 10.1). An alternative is to use the palm of the child's hand (not including the digits), if the area of the burn is small. This constitutes approximately 1% of the child's BSA.

Simple erythema should not be counted in the burn area.

Fluid requirements

The Parkland formula recommends *3–4 ml/kg/% body surface area of the burn*. Half of this volume should be given in the first eight hours following the burn and the remainder over the next 16 hours. This fluid is supplemented by the normal daily requirements of the child.

Additional fluids may be required, based upon indices of end organ perfusion. A urine output of at least 1 ml/kg/h is a useful guide.

Cardiovascular status, haematocrit and electrolyte balance will also guide fluid requirements.

Analgesia and dressings

Pain control should be instituted early. Intravenous morphine is ideal and should be given in small aliquots titrated to the pain.

Clingfilm acts as an ideal sterile, non-occlusive dressing which does not need removal to view the burns. Antibiotics, or topical preparations, should not be used unless there is a specific policy with the burns centre.

Children with burns are particularly susceptible to hypothermia. Measures to minimise heat loss

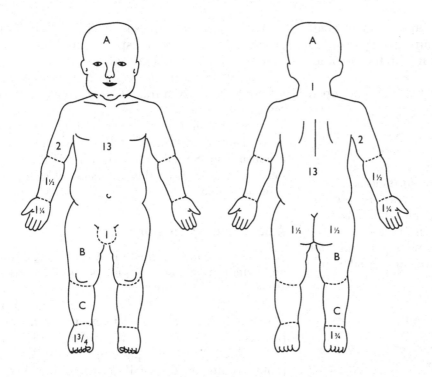

Figure 10.1 Calculation of body surface area (see Table 10.1 for percentages of different areas at different ages).

Table 10.1   Calculations of body surface area

Area %	Age (years)				
	0	1	5	10	15
A	9·5	8·5	6·5	5·5	4·5
B	2·75	3·25	4	4·5	4·5
C	2·5	2·5	2·75	3	3·25

must be instituted prior to transfer. Cold soaks are useful only in the first 20 minutes after a burn, and will exacerbate hypothermia after this time.

Practical procedures

Spinal immobilisation

Indications

The mechanism of injury suggests that injury to the cervical and/or thoracolumbar spinal column may have occurred. Cervical spine injuries constitute in excess of 95% of all spinal injuries in children.

Technique

Cervical spine immobilisation can be carried out by either:

- Manual inline immobilisation (Fig. 10.2) or
- Use of a hard collar, sandbags, and tape (bolsters and straps).

Manual immobilisation is labour intensive and requires some skill, but is useful when log rolling the patient and examining the neck. It is also useful in the irritable patient who is moving excessively, by allowing better cervical spine immobilisation in relation to the trunk.

The hard collar technique has three components, all of which must be present for adequate cervical spine immobilisation. However, the collar must be properly fitting in order to function optimally.

Log rolling the patient

Indications

- Examination of the patient's occiput, back, thoracolumbar spine, and the back of the legs.

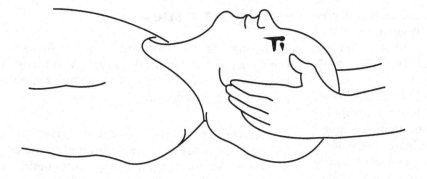

Figure 10.2 Manual cervical stabilisation.

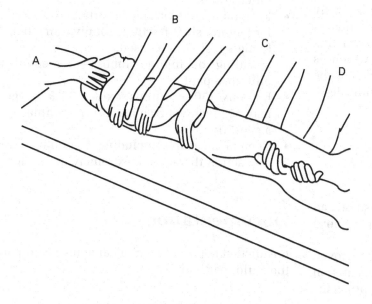

Figure 10.3 Log rolling—position of the team. (Adapted from Advanced Life Support Group. *Advanced Paediatric Life Support*, 3rd edn. London: BMJ Books, 2001.)

- Also allows removal of debris, broken glass, etc., on which the patient may be lying.
- Safe transfer onto or off the spinal board or vacuum mattress.

Technique (Fig. 10.3)

- Log rolling is a disciplined procedure. It requires each member of the team to know his or her role.
- It is essential, if possible, to explain to the patient what is going to happen. Give adequate analgesia prior to the log roll if necessary.
- For a small child (for example, age < 8 years) three persons are required to hold the patient while a fourth performs the examination. All should be clear about their roles.

Person A: Leads the log roll and holds the head and shoulders. Remember not to cover the child's ears—producing deafness will only increase anxiety.

Person B: Places one hand behind the patient's opposite shoulder and the other just above the pelvis.

Person C: Places one hand just below the pelvis and the other just below the opposite knee.

For larger children (for example, age > 8 years), four persons are required to hold the patient while a fifth performs the examination.

Person A: Leads the log roll and holds the head and shoulders.

Person B: Places one hand behind the patient's opposite shoulder and the other just above the pelvis.

Person C: Places one hand just below the pelvis and the other just above the opposite knee.

Person D: Places one hand just below the opposite knee and the other below the opposite ankle, maintaining that ankle level with the hip so as to minimise any abnormal movement of the lumbar spine.

Confirm that the team are aware of the degree to which the patient will be tilted (60° or 90°) and what the exact command is to start the roll (for example, "on 3", "after 3", "when I say roll", etc., etc.).

The person holding the head is in charge (team leader) and coordinates a smooth, slow, inline log roll, ensuring the patient's nose remains aligned with the umbilicus. After examination, the team leader coordinates a smooth log roll back to the supine position, and replaces hard collar, sandbags, and tape.

Make sure that the examining doctor carefully inspects the back of the scalp as well. A child can lose a significant proportion of their circulating volume from an occipital laceration which is missed. A rectal examination should not be performed in children unless strongly indicated.

Use of spinal boards and a vacuum mattress

Indications

- A spinal board is primarily of use as an extrication device in helping to remove patients from entrapped vehicles.
- The spinal board should be routinely removed after the primary survey and resuscitation phases. There are significant problems associated with prolonged use.
- The vacuum mattress should be considered the preferred spinal immobilisation transfer surface.

Splints

Splints act to control pain and prevent continuing haemorrhage from fractured long bones.

Indications

- Open or closed fractured limbs.
- Postreduction of dislocated joints.

A variety of splints are available.

- Plaster of Paris (POP) can be used to immobilise limbs not requiring traction.
- A variety of traction splints are available. The two commoner ones that are likely to be used for patient transport are the Hare and Sagar splints. Alternatively, skin traction with a Thomas splint may be used.

Analgesia issues

Analgesia is an essential part of safely transporting the injured child. A number of techniques are available which can be used either alone or in combination.

- Intravenous opiates. Morphine given intravenously in small aliquots titrated to the pain is the best form of analgesia. Antiemetics are not normally required on a prophylactic basis for children.
- Femoral nerve blockade is particularly suitable for femoral shaft fractures. Bupivacaine 0·25% (2 mg/kg) should be used.
- Splinting of injured limbs is essential to minimise pain.
- Entonox (50% nitrous oxide, 50% oxygen) may be given via face mask or mouthpiece for a short time.
- General measures including reassurance and distraction therapy are extremely important.

Documentation

Ensure that copies of all clinical notes accompany the child, particularly:

- Prehospital ambulance sheets
- All notes made by relevant specialty teams
- All blood test results
- Details of tetanus toxoid and immunoglobulin
- All blood transfusion records
- All original *x* ray films
- CT scans and results of other imaging modalities.

State clearly if specific diagnostic measures have not been completed, for example:

- Clearance of the spine
- Log rolling of the patient
- Completion of secondary survey for non-life threatening injuries to the upper and lower limbs.

There should be clear documentation detailing the senior doctor who has had responsibility for the child at the referring hospital as well as a contact name, phone number, and designated arrival point at the receiving hospital.

Pitfalls in the transfer of the injured child

The major principle of trauma management is to do no further harm. Care should consistently improve with each step, from the scene of the incident to the facility which can best provide the patient with the necessary definitive treatment.

Certain principles are especially important to ensure that this occurs.

Decision to transfer

Once the child has been stabilised and the need for transfer recognised, arrangements should not be delayed for *diagnostic procedures* that do not change the immediate plan.

However, review whether any other emergency *therapeutic procedures* need to be performed prior to transfer, for example fasciotomy for compartment syndrome, splinting of fractures, etc.

Ensure that the relevant specialties at the referring and receiving hospitals *communicate directly* with each other regarding ongoing trauma management.

Inadequate resuscitation

The child must not be transferred until adequately resuscitated and stabilised, otherwise transfer can be extremely hazardous with high morbidity and mortality rates.

Children usually have abundant physiological reserve and often demonstrate only subtle signs of hypovolaemia even after severe volume depletion. When deterioration does occur it is precipitous and catastrophic.

Evidence of adequate or enhanced end organ perfusion provides important evidence of satisfactory resuscitation, i.e. capillary refill, CNS status, and urinary output.

Monitoring

Ensure that all mandatory monitoring is functioning and that alarms are on.

When bradycardia occurs hypoxia must be excluded.

End tidal carbon dioxide ($ETco_2$) monitoring is mandatory for all intubated and ventilated patients, especially the head injured patient.

Remember that pulse oximetry does not measure ventilation or partial pressure of oxygen.

Central venous monitoring is optional. It can provide an indication of the response to fluid resuscitation, and may be particularly useful in the child with more than one body system injury. However, central vascular access should only be carried out by those expert in the technique.

Invasive blood pressure monitoring is strongly preferred.

Hypothermia

Reassess core temperature and minimise exposure of the child. Consider the use of an oesophageal temperature probe.

Ensure that measures to conserve body heat and rewarm the hypothermic child are enacted; for example, covering all burns, using warmed fluids and humidified oxygen, using warmed blankets.

Consider further active rewarming measures if indicated.

Summary

Prior to transport, the transport team must ensure that:

The PATIENT has had a primary and secondary trauma review performed and is clinically stable. All lines and tubes must be well secured

The PERSONNEL involved in the transport possess all the skills to deal with the transfer and those at the receiving hospital are fully aware of the patient's injuries

All PIECES of equipment, drugs and fluids required for the transport are maintained and fully functioning and present

All relevant documentation and PAPERWORK travel with the patient

The PARENTS or carers of the injured child are aware of the need for the transfer, and arrangements have been made for them to travel to the receiving hospital.

11 Special transport interventions

Objectives
The use of special transport modes will be
  discussed.
This will include the use of inhaled nitric oxide,
  nebulised prostacyclin, continuous positive
  airways pressure, prone ventilation, high
  frequency oscillation, and extracorporeal
  membrane oxygenation.

Inhaled nitric oxide

Background

Inhaled nitric oxide or iNO is in common use in
many paediatric and neonatal intensive care units.
It acts as a selective pulmonary vasodilator, which
can improve VQ matching in the lung, thereby
improving gas exchange. It also reduces
pulmonary artery pressure, which can be useful in
patients with congenital heart disease or persistent
fetal circulation. NO is made by pulmonary
vascular endothelium (and other tissues) when
L-arginine is cleaved by nitric oxide synthase
(NOS), releasing NO and citrulline. It has a half-
life in the circulation of around 6 seconds as it
immediately binds to haemoglobin to form met-
haemoglobin; this reduced form of haemoglobin
does not carry oxygen. NO stimulates the
intracellular production of cyclic GMP.

iNO in clinical practice

In clinical practice iNO is added to the ventilator
gases in a concentration of 5–20 ppm; this
improves oxygenation and has a moderate effect on
pulmonary artery pressure. iNO is proven to
reduce the need for extracorporeal membrane
oxygenation (ECMO) in term neonates (except
congenital diaphragmatic hernia); however, there
are no studies in any patient group which
demonstrate that iNO can reduce mortality. When
starting iNO it is usual to have an improvement
in oxygenation within a few minutes. Only
approximately 5% of neonates who do not
respond to 20 ppm iNO will have a response to
80 ppm. However, doses of around 80 ppm may
be needed if iNO is being used to treat pulmonary
hypertension. NOS is rapidly downregulated
when iNO is started, so that the patient's
endogenous NO production is greatly reduced.
In many patients this leads to severe rebound
pulmonary hypertension and hypoxia if iNO is
interrupted. Rebound can occur even in patients
who do not respond. It is therefore essential that all
patients who do not respond quickly have their
iNO stopped before downregulation of NOS occurs
(usually around 30 minutes). It is this rebound
phenomenon which makes mobile iNO necessary,
as patients who have received iNO for more than a
few hours will usually be unable to tolerate its
withdrawal during transport. In addition iNO is a
useful tool to improve the condition of a critically
hypoxic neonate. When taking the referral of a
patient who is receiving iNO it is essential to
establish if mobile iNO will be required. The
transporting team may ask the referring intensivist
to attempt to wean the iNO off and assess the
child's response. However, it is usually impossible
to withdraw iNO successfully, making retrieval on
the mobile iNO system necessary.

iNO set up for retrieval

The most suitable ventilators for iNO therapy are
those with a constant set gas flow. Ventilators
with variable flow are acceptable if the gas flow is
continuous, but those where the flow stops on
exhalation are unsuitable without bulky and
heavy iNO dosing apparatus.

A simple system (Fig. 11.1) is described below.

Delivery

A small gas cylinder (e.g. BOC's AZ size) is
adequate for around five hours' use at 20 ppm. It
should be fitted with a regulator to deliver low
pressure; about 0·5 bar is suitable. This feeds a
flowmeter of range approximately 0–500 l/min,
from which a line takes the set flow to the
ventilator circuit, well upstream of the patient to
allow good mixing. The required flow of gas can
be found from the formula:

$$\frac{\text{ppm NO required} \times \text{flow of gas in vent circuit}}{\text{ppm NO in cylinder}}$$

A "ready reckoner" is easy to make up, and handy
to decide the required gas flow quickly.

A useful refinement is to have a diverter valve
allowing the NO to be used in a bagging circuit.

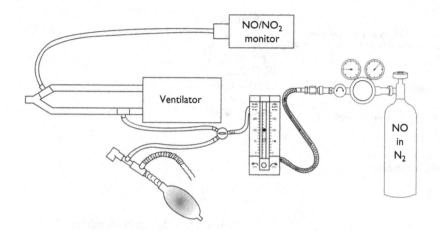

Figure 11.1 An iNO circuit. Note the position of the monitoring point next to the Y-piece. This may be on the inspiratory or expiratory limbs near to the Y-piece—where to measure from is largely a matter of convenience, using the existing breaks in the circuit. In practice, on our transport circuit, we deliver NO to a connector at the beginning of the inspiratory limb and measure from a port in the Y-piece.

Otherwise the whole line can be moved to a bag for manual ventilation if required.

Monitoring

Gas should be sampled from near the patient Y-piece. A monitor with a pump is preferred, since these have less trouble with water trapping in the line.

Scavenging

Since retrieval episodes are relatively short, and the air on most roads rich in oxides of nitrogen, scavenging may be regarded as optional. However, NO absorbing filters are available for the expiratory side of the vent if desired.

Leak monitoring

It is advisable to carry an environmental monitor in case of leaks arising between the cylinder and the flowmeter. Unlike the breathing gas, leaks of 1000 p.p.m. could present a hazard.

Safety requirements

Although a safe treatment when used correctly, iNO therapy has some inherent hazards. It is important that the retrieval team are fully trained and experienced in its use.

Nitrogen dioxide

NO oxidises to toxic NO_2 in oxygen. The industrial safe limit for NO_2 inhalation is 5 ppm; the clinical limit is 2 ppm. To minimise NO_2 exposure, it is very important to purge the NO delivery system

thoroughly by running it at high flow for a couple of minutes before connecting it to the patient circuit. Once running, NO_2 usually settles at 0·2 ppm or below.

Accidental leaks

Should the environmental monitor go off, check all fittings between the cylinder and the flowmeter immediately. But note that these monitors give false alarms in the presence of hydrocarbons, for example, from the ambulance exhaust, alcohol wipes, etc. NO_2 has a distinctive harsh metallic smell.

Interruption of NO to patient

When a patient has become NO dependent, their O_2 saturation drops rapidly if iNO is removed. It is important to carry enough gas, and have all lines secure. It is easy to forget that iNO must be switched over to the hand ventilation circuit in the heat of resuscitation.

Methaemoglobin

This may rise during iNO therapy, and should be monitored; however, this is rarely a consideration during transport.

In-flight use

The Civil Aviation Authority does not allow iNO to be used in civilian aircraft in the UK. However, no such prohibition exists for military aircraft and iNO has been used extensively in RAF Sea-King helicopters. Since the Sea-King is fairly draughty and has a large side door that can be opened in

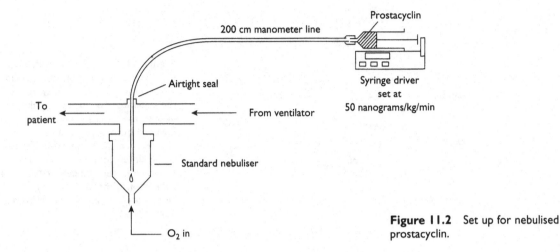

Figure 11.2 Set up for nebulised prostacyclin.

flight, it would be possible to provide good ventilation to the cabin space in the event of a cylinder leak. We do not believe that iNO has been used in a fixed wing aircraft in the UK.

Results of mobile iNO use

In a series of 55 paediatric and neonatal patients transported on iNO over a 1·5 year period, 19 were moved by helicopter and 36 by road. The Pao_2 improved from a mean pretransport value of 7·23 kPa (SD 5·26) to a mean level of 11·23 kPa (SD 7·32); there were no deaths or critical incidents.

Nebulised prostacyclin

Background

Prostacyclin or prostaglandin I_2 is in routine clinical use as an IV vasodilator and antiplatelet agent. It has a half-life of around two minutes and so is usually given as a continuous infusion. It is a non-selective vasodilator and will cause pulmonary and systemic vasodilatation if given IV. In higher doses IV prostacyclin can cause marked systemic hypotension. In common with all IV vasodilators, prostacyclin tends to dilate the perfused segments of lung and can therefore worsen VQ mismatch. However, administering the prostacyclin by nebuliser circumvents these limitations, as the drug is delivered to the ventilated segments, thereby improving VQ matching. Systemic absorption is also reduced, making systemic hypotension less of a problem.

Indications

Nebulised prostacyclin may be helpful in patients who will not wean from iNO or in critically hypoxic patients if mobile iNO is unavailable.

Administration

An inline nebuliser is placed in the inspiratory limb of the ventilator circuit. Oxygen is connected to the nebuliser and the flow rate adjusted according to the child's weight and lung compliance. Obviously the flow must be high enough to cause nebulisation, usually around 5 l/min. It may be necessary to reduce the flow rate from the transport ventilator to offset the nebuliser flow. A 50 ml syringe of prostacyclin is prepared according to the manufacturer's instruction (500 micrograms in 50 ml of the buffered diluent) and placed in a syringe driver. A 200 cm manometer line is connected to the syringe and primed, the manometer line is then introduced so that the drug enters the reservoir of the nebuliser (Fig. 11.2). The syringe gun is then set to deliver a dose of 50 nanograms/kg/min (this is about 10 times the IV dose).

Continuous positive airways pressure

Continuous positive airways pressure (CPAP) is widely used in neonatal intensive care. Although predominantly used as a weaning tool, a growing number of units are investigating the role of CPAP in conjunction with a developmentally supportive care regimen as the primary mode of

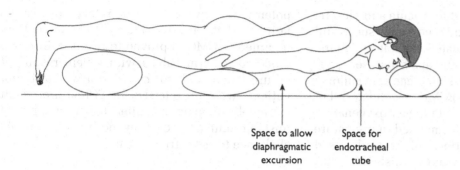

Space to allow
diaphragmatic
excursion

Space for
endotracheal
tube

Figure 11.3 Position of patient
for transfer during prone
ventilation.

respiratory support for many infants who might traditionally have been intubated and ventilated. Intubation is used to give surfactant if indicated, but with rapid extubation to CPAP. Good results appear possible with this approach to neonatal intensive care, which is widely practised in Scandinavia. Anecdotally its use is increasing in situations where infants would normally be intubated and ventilated for transfer.

CPAP may be delivered from a conventional ventilator using a short nasal tube or a proprietary CPAP device (INCA, Ackrad Laboratories, NJ, USA). The EME infant-flow CPAP driver (EME, Brighton, UK) is also available in a battery driven version that is suitable for transport, though its gas consumption is considerable and may be problematical on long transfers.

More research is needed on the risks and benefits of using CPAP in transport of acutely ill newborn infants.

Prone ventilation

Background

Prone positioning is in increasing use in adult and paediatric intensive care as a tool to improve VQ matching in patients with adult respiratory distress syndrome (ARDS) and pneumonia. These patients develop consolidation in the dependent posterior portions of their lungs as they lie supine. Turning them prone can result in improved VQ matching by redirecting blood flow to the now dependent anterior portions of the lungs. In addition there may be improved recruitment in the consolidated posterior area. Many patients experience an improvement in oxygenation when turned prone, but there is as yet no evidence demonstrating improved outcome. Better oxygenation and lung mechanics have also been demonstrated in neonates, both

ventilated and unventilated, when cared for in the prone position.

Indications

Some patients become unstable when they are turned back to the supine position. It may be necessary to transport these patients in the prone position.

Risks, benefits, and precautions

The prone position makes access to the airway impossible and makes external cardiac massage difficult. It is therefore essential to establish that the level of instability when the patient is turned supine would preclude transport; in other words that the risks of the prone position are outweighed by the benefits of being able to move the patient. Extra care must be given to the security of the endotracheal or tracheostomy tube as well as the central venous and arterial lines. Pillows are arranged transversely on the stretcher to cushion the patient's head, chest, pelvis, and knees. Gaps are left between the pillows for the endotracheal tube, and to allow diaphragmatic excursion (Fig. 11.3). In newborn infants the security of umbilical lines must be very thoroughly checked before transfer in the prone position. If a line fell out, substantial blood loss could go unnoticed. The benefits and risks of prone ventilation for transported infants have not been investigated.

High frequency oscillation

Background

High frequency oscillatory ventilation (HFOV) is in widespread use in many neonatal and paediatric ICUs. HFOV reduces acute and chronic lung injury in neonates, and seems to be successful in older children with isolated respiratory failure, but not those with extrapulmonary disease. It has also been used more successfully than conventional ventilation in neonatal ECMO candidates, but seems ineffective in those with higher oxygenation indexes. HFOV is not recommended in premature infants outside the settings of a randomised controlled trial. There are no published studies demonstrating an improved outcome with HFOV.

HFOV is used in a "high-volume strategy" to recruit collapsed portions of lung, thereby reducing VQ mismatch and improving oxygenation. It is common practice to use a higher mean airway pressure on HFOV than during conventional ventilation, but because the sheer stress is eliminated (as there is no mass gas flow during HFOV) the amount of ventilator induced lung injury is reduced. Similar improvements in oxygenation have been achieved in the laboratory if a sufficiently high mean airway pressure and PEEP is used during conventional ventilation to achieve lung recruitment. Some children who are receiving HFOV do not tolerate the switch back to conventional ventilation, even when higher airway pressures are used. This may be due to haemodynamic instability or because of reduced CO_2 clearance.

Mobile HFOV

The VDR-3C (Percussionaire, Sandpoint, Idaho, USA) is a hybrid ventilator which can provide mobile HFOV. It has been used by a number of teams in the USA and Canada but is not yet available in the UK. Currently therefore there is no solution in the UK to the problem of transporting a child receiving HFOV who cannot be stabilised on conventional ventilation and iNO.

Mobile extracorporeal membrane oxygenation

Background

Extracorporeal membrane oxygenation, or ECMO, uses a modified cardiopulmonary bypass circuit to provide prolonged cardiorespiratory support in the ICU. It may be used for patients of any age from 34 weeks' gestation up to adulthood, with potentially reversible respiratory or cardiac failure that is refractory to conventional treatment. ECMO is proven to result in improved outcome in term babies with severe respiratory failure compared to conventional ventilation. Patients who are referred for ECMO are usually extremely hypoxic and often haemodynamically unstable and as such they pose a considerable challenge to the retrieval team.

Mobile ECMO

Despite the seeming instability of these patients the vast majority can be transported with a good outcome—in nearly 750 transports of neonates and children with severe respiratory and cardiac failure over a four year period there were no deaths during transport. However, it remains a concern when faced with the prospect of transporting an unstable patient with end stage cardiorespiratory failure. In order to address this problem a number of units have developed the capability to establish the patient on ECMO at the referring hospital. This facility is only used for the most unstable patients who are believed to be at greatest risk of death during transport. Despite this the survival in the group of patients who are retrieved on ECMO is usually better than that in patients who are transported conventionally.

Obviously the provision of mobile ECMO is a huge logistical exercise involving the participation of a large multidisciplinary team and the extensive use of resources. Mobile ECMO circuits in current use are very similar to those in hospital use, with the exception of the type of pump used. Whilst some systems use a standard servoregulated roller pump (in both neonates and adults), the majority use centrifugal pumps which are not in common use in hospitals. Centrifugal pumps are felt to be superior to roller pumps during mobile ECMO, as they are safer in the event of inflow or outlet obstruction. This means that they are less sensitive to acceleration and deceleration than roller pumps. The ability of a centrifugal pump to exert venous suction to improve venous drainage is a definite advantage during retrieval, when increasing the height of the bed above the pump cannot be used to increase the venous siphon. This same property causes haemolysis during prolonged hospital use of the centrifugal pump if the inlet pressure is not regulated. Mobile ECMO is currently under development in the UK and should be available for clinical use soon.

Summary

The most important factor in the decision to use special transport modes is the evaluation of the risk : benefit ratio between not transporting the patient and taking the risk of transport.

Tolerating a lower Pao_2 than normal, whilst ensuring adequate perfusion and a normal haematocrit, may allow you to transfer the patient to a centre for definitive care.

The use of permissive hypercapnia, often with the use of buffers, can allow transport with a conventional ventilator.

The ability to use iNO during transport is a great advantage but has not been shown to alter outcome.

Prone ventilation is useful in intensive care, but adds to the stress of transport for the operator, particularly in the larger child and adolescent.

12 What to do when it all goes wrong

Objectives
With adequate preparation and intervention, most retrievals will pass off without any problems. It has been demonstrated that even the sickest patients can be transferred safely if the accompanying staff have the appropriate training and equipment. However, sometimes things do go wrong, and some days it will seem as if *everything* is going wrong. The purpose of this chapter is to discuss some situations where problems may arise, and to suggest strategies for dealing with them.

Inappropriate referrals

There will be a small minority of referrals where the child does not appear to be "sick enough" for the intensive care unit (ICU). In this case it is important to ascertain that you have recorded the history accurately.

- Ask what particular features are giving the referring team concern, as this may help you to identify abnormal clinical signs or symptoms that you have missed.
- Is the referring physician of appropriate experience to assess the child? Referrals should ideally be made at consultant level.
- What is the workload and skill mix of the referring hospital? Is the child being referred on a Friday afternoon because staffing levels over the weekend mean that the hospital cannot maintain care for a "high dependency" patient.

In all cases it is important to maintain communication with the referring clinicians, whether or not the child is accepted for intensive care.

Very rarely the ICU will receive calls from practitioners in the community when an emergency ambulance is needed. First aid and basic life support advice should be given, but this should not delay a call to the ambulance service being made.

Referrals from a second source—for example, a plastic surgery registrar who accepts a child with burns and who then phones the paediatric intensive care unit (PICU) "for a bed"—should be discouraged, as there is no opportunity to give advice on stabilising the child, and important details may be lost or forgotten. In any case, the clinicians actually caring for the child at the time of the referral should be contacted for information directly.

Children referred inappropriately for the expertise of the unit—for example, referral of a head injury to a centre that doesn't have neurosurgery—should be referred on to a more appropriate centre. Some centres that provide retrieval services prefer to do this themselves, allowing the referring clinicians to spend more time stabilising the child.

Some children will improve before you arrive at the referring hospital, so that they no longer need intensive care. If there is any doubt, bring them back to the ICU, as the improvement may only be temporary.

Unsalvageable child

Occasionally you will arrive at the referring hospital to find that the patient has deteriorated in the interim and is now clearly not going to survive.

- How much intervention do you undertake?
- Do you scoop and run back to the intensive care unit, or do you withdraw intensive care at the referring centre?
- Should you retrieve patients just to "manage the death"? Or should the child stay at the referring centre who may know the family better?
- Does the amount of intervention given depend on the expectation of the referring team?

These are all very difficult questions that will depend on the local situation and the seniority of the retrieval team. It is impossible to be prescriptive and the following comments will not apply to all situations.

Both the family and the referring hospital will want to know that everything possible has been done for the child, and so a full assessment and aggressive treatment of immediately remediable problems should be undertaken. Therefore ensure that the airway is patent and that ventilation is adequate. Consider giving volume and inotropes.

Most importantly, discuss the situation with base, the referring clinicians, and the parents. Their expectations will guide you. An important aspect of the situation is that the parents may need time to "say goodbye", and to allow other relatives to be with the patient before he or she dies. Time to undertake religious ceremonies such as baptism may be needed. It is not an inappropriate use of an ICU bed to allow time for this to happen, either by bringing the child back to base, moving to an adult ICU in the referring hospital, or providing intensive care for a longer time than normal in the child's current location.

Some practitioners feel that transferring such children from a unit where they may know the staff to a regional ICU where they do not is unnecessary and unhelpful. Don't forget that transferring these children to "manage the death" imposes a significant emotional and psychological burden on your own staff.

The situation may be different if the child is referred to a specialist centre, for example, for extracorporeal membrane oxygenation or neurosurgery, where specialist intervention may be life saving.

The potential for organ donation should not be forgotten and should be discussed with the organ transplant team, the referring team and, where appropriate, with the parents. If organ donation is a possibility, intensive care will need to be continued.

Death in transit

This is fortunately rare, although there are only anecdotal data on its incidence. If a child arrests, and resuscitation is unsuccessful, a number of questions arise.

- *How long to continue resuscitation?* This will depend to some extent on the seniority of the escorting team. It can be very lonely in the back of an ambulance, and there will be very little peer support to help you decide that further resuscitation is futile. No hard and fast rules can be made. However, the same guidelines for continuing resuscitation in hospital apply in transit.
- *What is the diagnosis?* In hypothermia and some poisonings you may continue cardiopulmonary resuscitation (CPR) for a lot longer than normal.
- *Where are you going?* If you are transporting the child to a centre for a particular life saving therapy, it may be justified to continue for longer.
- *How far away are you from base, or an alternative hospital?* If you are close, continue until you arrive and can get help.

Nurse practitioners cannot certify death. A collapse during a transfer led by an advanced neonatal nurse practitioner mandates full resuscitation being continued until the baby is delivered to a medical team.

> *However long you continue for, remember two rules:*
> If you're doing CPR, make it *good* CPR.
> Any hospital is a better hospital than the back of an ambulance.

If the child dies in the back of the ambulance, it is best to go to wherever the parents are. If the parents are already on their way to your ICU, you should probably continue there to be with the parents. Alternatively you may need to return to the referring unit. Do not be misled by anecdotal concerns about place of death and county boundaries being the determining factors in where you should go to.

In general, deaths occurring during retrieval should be referred to the coroner. Depending on local policies, lines and endotracheal tubes should be left *in situ* until after discussion with the coroner.

Morbidity in transit

Previous studies have suggested a high level of untoward incidents during interhospital transport. Most of these related to equipment failure (often power related) or failure to recognise poor oxygenation and shock. Such incidents are reduced by appropriate training of staff, forward planning and familiarity with retrieval equipment.

Dealing with parents

It may be your fourth retrieval of the week, but for the parents and family of the child the situation is a unique, unforeseen crisis of immeasurable proportions. Not only is their son or daughter critically ill, but they are about to be taken on a dangerous journey to a distant hospital by complete strangers. The physical appearance of the child and the dramatic nature of the arrival of the retrieval team only heighten the parents' feelings that the child is in imminent danger.

Initially, parents go through a feeling of shock and disbelief, accompanied by helplessness.

Coping mechanisms at this stage may include aggression, regression, withdrawal, or repression. It is important that the retrieval team respond to these manifestations to enhance the parent's coping strategy. Thus verbal expressions of anger, guilt or animosity should be met with reassurance and acceptance. Emotional outbursts may be expected, and reassurance that the child is being appropriately cared for and comforted can reduce parental anxiety.

Parents need information about their child, and they need to know that the retrieval team care for the child as an individual in his or her own right. Therefore make time to speak privately to the parents. Make sure that you know the child's name, and give the parents the opportunity to express their fears and ask questions.

The parents will remember little of what is said to them at this stage. Give the most important information first, and summarise it at the end of the discussion. Be realistic and do not be afraid to say that you do not know the answers to certain questions. Be careful not to undermine the care given by the team at the referring hospital.

Loss of physical control for the wellbeing of their child is a major stress for the parents. This may be reduced by allowing them access to the child during the stabilisation phase. Typically, one of the staff from the referring team may be allocated to explain to the parents what is being done and why. Other major stresses are seeing the child in pain or frightened, seeing the child unable to communicate, and not knowing how best to protect the child.

In most cases, it is not possible for the parents to travel with the child on the return journey to the intensive care unit. Separate transport should be arranged, or they need to be given specific directions to the hospital, information on parking, and directions to get to the intensive care unit. They should be discouraged from trying to follow the ambulance.

Debriefing and staff support

Intensive care is by its very nature stressful, and transporting very sick children in a strange and hostile environment, isolated from normal support, may lead to a great deal of anxiety in the retrieval team.

Improvements occur following reflective practice and structured debriefing that allow the team to identify aspects of the retrieval that have gone well, and those that have lead to problems or potential problems. These debriefings should be non-judgemental and may be best facilitated by a psychologist or appropriately trained counsellor.

Structures exist in both the medical and nursing professions for dealing with concerns about poor staff performance. Initially these should be addressed in private with the person concerned by their mentor, line manager, or the unit's retrieval coordinator.

Audit and critical incident monitoring

Monitoring the quality and effectiveness of the care delivered during the retrieval process is fundamental to the delivery of a high quality transport service. Information is needed not only on utilisation of the service, to enable future planning, but also on management aspects of each retrieval to identify features that characterise the optimum retrieval and those which need improvement or change. Reflection and review of each retrieval in a semistructured forum will also be educational for staff and trainees. Transport always happens in isolation, and is often a powerful learning experience for the individuals involved. The purpose of these sessions is to allow the whole team access to these experiences, so that the learning is shared.

Accurate information gathering is paramount to the success of a quality improvement programme. For this reason, data collection should be made as easy as possible, and should be organised so that data collectors not only know the relevance of the forms they are being asked to complete, but also have a vested interest in ensuring that they are completed accurately. Checks should be built in to the system to provide information on the data accuracy and feedback to the staff.

Review meetings may be held regularly to feedback to staff about changes in the retrieval service, administrative issues, performance indicators, and also to go through specific retrievals to highlight areas where there have been problems.

Critical incident monitoring is essential to the running of an intensive care service. Mistakes happen and problems occur primarily because of a fault with the system (whether it be in training, communication, or a specific fault with equipment) rather than a fault with individuals.

For this reason, critical incident monitoring should be anonymous and non-judgemental.

Transport services should have robust incident reporting procedures to pick up when there has been a serious problem or near miss during a journey. In most cases these should be used as a learning tool rather than a disciplinary matter. In particular, other members of the transport team should hear about the problem so that they can learn from the key features of the incident so that they might respond appropriately should the same thing happen to them.

As far as we are aware, there is no mechanism for the accreditation and training of intensive care staff in paediatric and neonatal critical care transport. In-house training, evaluation and accreditation is therefore of importance. Courses such as the Neonatal Life Support course and the Advanced Paediatric Life Support course will give practitioners many of the skills in specific aspects of caring for a patient during interhospital transfer.

Severity of illness and scoring systems

Reference has already been made to the Glasgow Coma Scale. Other scoring systems are also useful for prognostication and for audit. The Glasgow Meningococcal Septicaemia Prognostic Score (GMSPS) is a specific risk of mortality score for meningococcal septicaemia (Table 12.1). In one series a score of 9 or more had a specificity of 95% and a positive predictive value for death of 74%.

Other severity of illness scores, such as the Paediatric Risk of Mortality (PRISM) score or the Paediatric Index of Mortality (PIM) score, may be used as audit tools. Both of these scores use the data collected from the first contact of the intensive care team with the patient, rather than the physical admission of the child to the PICU, so it is important to collect accurate data from the time of arrival at the referring hospital. The neonatal retrieval forms in Appendix 1 show how

Table 12.1 Glasgow Meningococcal Septicaemia Prognostic Score

Risk factor	Score
Systolic BP (< 75 mmHg age < 4 years, < 85 mmHg age > 4 years)	3
Core/peripheral temperature gap > 3°C	3
Modified Coma Scale < 8, or deterioration of ≥ 3 points in 1 hour	3
Deterioration in clinical condition in the hour before scoring	2
Absence of meningism	2
Extending purpuric rash, or widespread ecchymoses	1
Base deficit ≥ 8·0 (arterial or capillary)	1
Maximum score	15

a transport score can be used to easily collect readily available data at critical points on a transfer.

A number of transport teams use intervention records or intervention scores such as the Therapeutic Intervention Scoring System (TISS) to quantify the medical and nursing activity during transfer. Typically, intervention scores increase prior to transfer as the retrieval team intubate, cannulate and catheterise to ensure a smooth run home.

Summary
With prior preparation, a sound knowledge of the equipment used, and good clinical skills, most retrievals should occur without incident.
Occasionally difficult clinical, administrative and ethical problems arise that would tax the skills of most of us. Forethought and prior discussion within the retrieval team will help you deal with these, and advice from colleagues at your base hospital during the retrieval is invaluable.
Finally, after the dust has settled, revisit the problem with your colleagues and determine how to deal with it next time.

13 Drugs

To be able to practise safely, a sound knowledge of the pharmacology of drugs that are commonly used in intensive care is vital.

> **Objectives**
> To know the dose, effects and side effects of the drugs commonly used when transferring critically ill patients between hospitals.
> To understand some of the practical issues in the administration of those drugs.
> To be able to prescribe and administer intravenous fluid therapy appropriately.
> To remember that neonates handle drugs differently.

The following are the common groups of drugs that are relevant to the care of the critically ill child and neonate:

- Analgesics
- Sedatives
- Muscle relaxants
- Vasoactive drugs
- Steroids
- Anticonvulsants
- Antiarrhythmics
- Antihypertensives
- Neonatal respiratory drugs.

Each group will be discussed, giving the onset and duration of action, the dose, the main side effects and any critical issues involved in the administration of the particular agent.

As with all textbooks and guidelines, the reader has the responsibility to ensure that the drugs and dosages given here are appropriate for any particular patient. Although we have checked these carefully, no responsibility can be taken for any errors that have slipped through. The reader should become familiar with the use of a few key drugs, many of which are discussed below.

Analgesics

The control of pain is one of the most important functions of the team looking after a critically ill child. The ability of neonates and infants to feel pain has been poorly recognised in the past and has led to inadequate treatment.

The aim of providing analgesia and sedation is to provide hypnosis and pain relief, and to reduce the normal sympathetic response to various noxious stimuli, as well as leaving the patient with as little memory of the episode as possible. Sedation and analgesia also help to slow down metabolism in a sick and agitated child as well as promote more efficient breathing. Transported ventilated infants and children should routinely receive pain relief and sedation.

The most commonly used analgesics are the opiates. Of this group, the two most frequently used are morphine and fentanyl.

Morphine

Provides excellent analgesia and sedation.

Onset of action: 5 minutes.

Duration of action: 3–5 hours.

Dose: As a bolus, 0·1–0·2 mg/kg IV. As an infusion, 5–40 micrograms/kg/h. Infusion for neonates: 5–10 micrograms/kg/h.

Side effects: Respiratory depression.

Neonates are more sensitive to morphine as the immature blood–brain barrier allows more drug to penetrate into the brain. In addition, it is cleared less predictably and more slowly in the neonate, predisposing to higher drug levels.

It also causes reduced gastric and intestinal motility, nausea, vomiting, and pruritus. In addition, morphine is vagotonic and may cause bradycardia.

Critical issues: Equipment to support the airway must be on hand while administering opiates to critically ill patients. If its antagonist naloxone is administered to combat respiratory depression, the analgesic effect is also reversed and that needs to be addressed.

Morphine is associated with histamine release, which is detrimental to a hypotensive patient or an asthmatic. Use boluses of morphine with care and have fluid drawn up to administer if necessary.

Morphine can be administered IV, IM, or SC.

Fentanyl

Is more potent than morphine but shorter acting.

Onset of action: Almost immediate.

Duration of action: 30–60 minutes.

Dose: As a bolus, 1–5 micrograms/kg IV slowly. As an infusion, 1–10 micrograms/kg/h.

Side effects: Like morphine but causes less histamine release. Doses above 15 micrograms/kg are associated with chest wall rigidity and will need muscle relaxants to be administered simultaneously.

Critical issues: As it is associated with less histamine release, it is "cardiovascularly" stable and is commonly used for cardiovascular anaesthesia. It can also be used in bronchial asthma. Not widely used in neonatal intensive care, due to the side effect profile and serious withdrawal symptoms.

Ketamine

An intravenous anaesthetic agent with powerful analgesic properties.

It is one of the most commonly used IV anaesthetics prior to intubation, be it rapid sequence intubation or elective. Its effects on the blood pressure are either to cause no change or to cause an elevation in the blood pressure. It is therefore one of the anaesthetics of choice in the setting of hypovolaemia and hypertension.

Onset of action: Almost immediate.

Duration of action: 5–10 minutes.

Dose: 1–2 mg/kg as an IV bolus.

Side effects: It can cause an increase intracranial pressure hence is contraindicated in pathological states of raised intracranial pressure. It can also lower the seizure threshold and should be used with caution in status epilepticus.

Critical issues: It can be given intramuscularly if there is no IV access.

Also ketamine is associated with post-anaesthetic emergence reactions such as dreams, hallucinations, nightmares. These side effects are minimised by pretreatment with benzodiazepines.

Not widely used in neonatal intensive care.

Thiopentone

Short acting barbiturate which is used as an intravenous anaesthetic and an anticonvulsant.

It is the drug of choice for anaesthetising a patient with raised intracranial pressure for rapid sequence intubation. It can also be used as a continuous infusion in refractory status epilepticus.

Onset of action: Almost immediate.

Duration of action: 5–30 minutes.

Dose: 2–4 mg/kg IV.

Side effects: Rapid IV injection can cause hypotension. Higher doses can cause myocardial depression.

Critical issues: Reduces cerebral metabolism, hence used in raised intracranial pressure. Higher doses can cause loss of pupillary reactions. Not widely used in neonatal intensive care.

Sedatives

Critically ill children are usually also very anxious and frightened. Therefore apart from providing analgesia it is equally important to administer sedatives to provide reduction of anxiety, sedation, and amnesia, and in many situations to provide an anticonvulsant effect.

The most commonly used IV sedatives are the benzodiazepines.

Midazolam

Currently the most commonly used IV sedative.

Onset of action: 1–5 minutes.

Duration of action: 30–45 minutes.

Dose: 0·1–0·2 mg/kg IV as a bolus. Doses up to 0·5 mg/kg may be used.

Can be used as an intravenous infusion in the dose of 1–10 micrograms/kg/min. In newborns, start at 1 microgram/kg/min. In infants less than 33 weeks' gestation this dose must be halved after 24 hours to prevent drug accumulation and the possibility of encephalopathic illness.

Side effects: Can cause respiratory depression but that is seen more often when used concomitantly with opiates. Hypotension especially if administered rapidly. Withdrawal and dependence.

Treatment of overdose is with flumazenil.

Critical issues: Midazolam is a very good anticonvulsant and can be used as an infusion in spontaneously breathing patients to provide sedation or an anticonvulsant effect. Causes less respiratory depression than diazepam.

Diazepam

Currently its main use in the ICU setting is as an anticonvulsant.

Onset of action: 1–3 minutes.

Duration of action: May be > 24 hours

Dose: 0·1–0·2 mg/kg IV.

Side effects: Respiratory depression is relatively common when given as a rapid IV push. Can be caustic on veins. Hypotension due to reduction in peripheral vascular resistance and venous return.

Critical issues: If the patient becomes apnoeic supporting the patient with bag-valve-mask ventilation for a few minutes is often adequate rather than jumping in and intubating the patient. Rarely used in neonatal intensive care.

Lorazepam

Recent addition to the selection of clinically useful sedatives.

Onset of action: 4–10 minutes.

Duration of action: 4–6 hours.

Dose: 0·05–0·1 mg/kg IV as a bolus. 25 micrograms/kg/h as an IV infusion.

Side effects: Similar to other benzodiazepines.

Critical issues: Good anticonvulsant and causes less respiratory depression than diazepam.

APLS guidelines suggest using lorazepam as the first line anticonvulsant. Rarely used in neonatal intensive care.

Muscle relaxants

Are used more commonly in paediatric intensive care than in adult or neonatal intensive care.

Broadly, there are three situations for use of muscle relaxants.

1. For rapid sequence intubation (RSI) in a child who is rapidly deteriorating regardless of the underlying pathology.
2. For semielective intubation in a child with potential respiratory failure, who is steadily worsening. In general, suxamethonium is the muscle relaxant of choice in this situation (see below).
3. To allow artificial ventilation to proceed in an infant or child who is "fighting" the ventilator.

For infants and children in whom you wish to maintain muscle relaxation for transfer, choose an agent such as atracurium that may be given

by infusion. When using muscle relaxants as continuous infusions, the team caring for the child must regularly reassess the indication for the drug and monitor the depth of paralysis.

It is also of paramount importance to ensure that while a child is paralysed, he/she has adequate sedation/analgesia. In addition, remember that although a child cannot overtly fit when paralysed, they may still actually be fitting.

Muscle relaxants should never be given unless it has been demonstrated that it is possible to support the breathing by bag-valve-mask ventilation.

Suxamethonium

Onset of action: 30–60 seconds.

Duration of action: 5–7 minutes.

Dose: 1–3 mg/kg IV.

Side effects: Painful muscle fasciculation (give sedative first). Anaphylaxis. Malignant hyperpyrexia. Cardiac arrhythmias, especially bradycardia. Myoglobinaemia, myoglobinuria, masseter spasm, and a rise in intragastric and intraocular pressure.

Pretreatment with atropine may reduce the incidence of bradycardia.

Critical issues: Serum potassium levels may become dangerously elevated following suxamethonium administration in children with burns, massive trauma, major neurological disease, and renal failure. Could lead to hyperkalaemic arrest. Contraindicated in severe liver disease.

Can be given intramuscularly (1–2 mg/kg IM) if no IV access available, but you need to be very certain of your competence before paralysing a child without IV access. If necessary, put in an intraosseous needle.

Prolonged paralysis may occur in patients with low plasma pseudocholinesterase, and with repeated doses of suxamethonium.

Atracurium

A non-steroid based muscle relaxant. Used in rapid sequence intubation where there is a contraindication to suxamethonium. May be given as infusion for maintaining muscle relaxation during transfer.

Onset of action: 2–5 minutes.

Duration of action: 30–40 minutes.

Dose: 0·3–0·5 mg/kg as a bolus. In RSI, higher doses up to 1 mg/kg may be used to give a quicker onset of paralysis. 10–40 micrograms/kg/min as a continuous infusion. Neonates start at 6–8 micrograms/kg/min.

Side effects: Said to be associated with histamine release. May rarely drop blood pressure or worsen bronchospasm. May cause flushing, urticaria, and pruritus.

Critical issues: It is metabolised by the endothelial cells by a process of Hoffman degradation. Therefore it is the drug of choice in hepatorenal impairment.

Atracurium is not the drug of choice for rapid sequence intubation as it might take 2–5 minutes to paralyse the child.

Recently, a stereoisomer of atracurium has been released called *cis*-atracurium. It is more potent than atracurium and is associated with less histamine release. It is therefore the muscle relaxant of choice in bronchial asthma.

Pancuronium

Steroid based muscle relaxant.

Onset of action: 2–5 minutes.

Duration of action: 40–60 minutes.

Dose: 0·05–0·1 mg/kg as a bolus and 0·1 mg/kg as required.

Side effects: Has gone out of favour recently because of the associated tachycardia.

Vecuronium

Steroid based muscle relaxant. Good cardiovascular profile.

Onset of action: 1–3 minutes.

Duration of action: 30–40 minutes.

Dose: 0·1 mg/kg as a bolus. 1–10 micrograms/kg/min as a continuous infusion.

Side effects: As it is a steroid based compound, its long-term use has been associated with prolonged muscle weakness. Accumulates in cases of hepatorenal impairment.

Rocuronium

A recent introduction, without the side effect profile of suxamethonium.

Onset of action: Less than 60 seconds.

Duration of action: 30–40 minutes.

Dose: For rapid onset of action, 1·2 mg/kg as a bolus.

Side effects: No long term studies available but has fewer side effects than suxamethonium.

Critical issues: Can be given intramuscularly as well. It has a longer duration of action than suxamethonium.

Vasoactive drugs

Cardiac dysfunction is relatively common in the critically ill child. After restoring intravascular volume, attention must be paid to supporting the pump. In various disease states, for example sepsis, it is common to have circulating molecules that act as myocardial depressants.

Vasoactive drugs increase the heart rate when it is inappropriately slow for the clinical condition and increase the contractility of the heart, thereby increasing cardiac output. The most commonly used drugs are sympathomimetic agents that stimulate adrenergic receptors. Receptor activation is different with each drug and can change with varying doses to produce diverse cardiovascular effects.

Vasoactive drugs should be titrated to provide maximal therapeutic effects with minimal side or toxic effects.

Neonates depend more on their heart rate than stroke volume for their cardiac output.

Receptors

* *Alpha*, when stimulated, lead to constriction of arterioles and veins, thereby increasing afterload.
* *Beta*$_1$ are associated with an increased contractility as well as an increase in heart rate and conduction velocity.
* *Beta*$_2$ are associated with peripheral vasodilatation and bronchodilatation.
* *Dopaminergic* are associated with an increase in renal and splanchnic blood flow.

Dopamine

Is a naturally occurring catecholamine.

Dose: 3–5 micrograms/kg/min: stimulates dopamine receptors in the renal vessels, increasing renal blood flow and causing an increase in urine output.

5–10 micrograms/kg/min: causes stimulation of beta-receptors (beta$_1$-receptors) and an increase in myocardial contractility.

10–20 micrograms/kg/min: beta-receptor stimulation persists but alpha-receptor activation starts to appear and increases with increasing doses. The alpha effects will lead to constriction of blood vessels, leading to hepatic and mesenteric ischaemia, an increase in the work of the heart and an increase in oxygen consumption.

Side effects: Tachycardia, tachyarrhythmias, and pulmonary vasoconstriction.

Critical issues: Tissue necrosis can occur following extravasation if not administered via a central line. Dopamine has a very short half-life and needs to be administered by a continuous infusion.

Dobutamine

Is a synthetic catecholamine with different effects on receptors.

Dose: 5–20 micrograms/kg/min: selective beta effects with an increase in cardiac contractility and a variable increase in heart rate.
Beta$_2$ effects produce mild peripheral vasodilatation.
No dopaminergic or alpha effects seen.

Side effects: Can cause tachyarrhythmia although less common than with dopamine.

Critical issues: Can be given peripherally and can therefore be used early on in a child with low cardiac output.
Due to afterload reducing effects, is useful in a child with myocardial failure.

Epinephrine (adrenaline)

Powerful inotrope with both alpha and beta effects.

Dose: 0·05–0·2 micrograms/kg/min beta$_1$ effects predominate; > 0·5 micrograms/kg/min alpha effects predominate.

Side effects: The alpha effects can lead to an increase in myocardial work and oxygen consumption and constriction of renal and splanchnic vesssels. Can lead to tachyarrhythmias.

Critical issues: As it is a powerful inotrope, should be considered relatively early in patients with refractory hypotension.

Should be infused through a central line due to extravasation tissue necrosis.

Other situations in which it is used are anaphylactic shock, asystolic arrest, as a bronchodilator in asthma and acute bronchiolitis, and nebulised as a mucosal vasoconstrictor in croup.

Norepinephrine (noradrenaline)

Powerful vasoconstrictor.

Dose: 0·1–1 microgram/kg/min. It has more potent alpha than beta effects.

Side effects: Similar to epinephrine (adrenaline). Main problem is potent alpha effects.

Critical issues: Useful in refractory shock due to profound vasodilatation.
Renal vasoconstriction can be partly overcome by concomitant use of dopamine in renal doses.

Isoprenaline

Used in very selected situations, mainly for its chronotropic effect.

Dose: 0·05–1·5 micrograms/kg/min beta$_1$ and beta$_2$ effects. Significant chronotropy, i.e. increase in heart rate.

Side effects: Will increase myocardial oxygen consumption and may cause tachyarrhythmias.

Critical issues: Can be used peripherally. Useful in neonates and infants where heart rate is inappropriately low. Also used to treat heart block.

Enoximone

Non-adrenergic inotrope that leads to phosphodiesterase inhibition and ultimately an increase in available calcium. This results in improved cardiac contractility and significant vasodilatation.

Dose: 5–20 micrograms/kg/min.

Side effects: May cause arrhythmias and hypotension, especially if the patient is hypovolaemic.

Critical issues: Has to be administered on its own, but can be administered through one lumen of a central line. As it is an inodilator, it is commonly used in children with chronic heart failure or myocarditis. Have a fluid bolus drawn up and ready to administer in case of hypotension.

Steroids

A very controversial issue. Steroids were widely used in newborns to assist weaning from ventilation and oxygen, but recent evidence of their effects on neurodevelopment and growth has led to a re-examination of this strategy. Steroid use should be strictly limited in the neonatal intensive care unit and they will not normally be needed on transport.

In septic states steroids act in a number of ways, an important one being by reducing cytokine levels. The crucial issue is the timing of the steroid, i.e. it should be administered before the cytokine levels reach a critical amount. Studies that have shown steroids to be effective recommend that they be given before the first dose of antibiotic, which would cause cytokine liberation on cell death, and lysis of the cell wall. Are also useful in states of massive inflammation such as bronchial asthma, croup.

Dose: Methylprednisolone 10–30 mg/kg/day.
   Dexamethasone: 0·1–0·5 mg/kg/dose 6 hourly.

Side effects: Hypertension, hyperglycaemia, leucocytosis. Other long term side effects are well documented, but not normally relevant to patient transport.

Critical issues: Studies have shown that high doses of steroids are associated with increased mortality. That has not been shown to be the case for more conventional doses; in fact, recent literature suggests a possible beneficial effect of low dose steroids in children with hyperinflammatory states like sepsis even if given after the first dose of antibiotics.

Anticonvulsants

Stabilisation of the airway, breathing and circulation are the first priority in treating convulsions. Pharmacological management should be initiated during stabilisation. Apart from using anticonvulsants, serum calcium, magnesium and blood sugar must always be routinely monitored and aggressively corrected if abnormal.

A sequential approach to seizure management is preferred.

The benzodiazepines (lorazepam, midazolam, and diazepam) are the drugs most commonly used for acute termination of the seizure. Sometimes a second drug will be required for acute and long term management of the seizures.

In the newborn, phenobarbitone is most frequently used as the first anticonvulsant with paraldehyde and clonazepam used subsequently.

Refer to local policy for details of seizure management in practice.

Since the drugs are associated with respiratory depression, equipment and personnel capable of managing the airway should be present.

Phenobarbitone

Increases the levels of GABA which is the main inhibitory neurotransmitter in the brain.

Dose: Loading dose of 20 mg/kg at a rate not faster than 1 mg/kg/min IV.

Subsequent doses: Newborns: 10 mg/kg 30–60 minutes after the loading dose if fitting continues, up to 30–40 mg/kg total dose.
   Older children: Can be given in stepwise progression up to a maximum of 60 mg/kg. Maintenance dose 5–8 mg/kg/day.

Side effects: Can cause drowsiness. Increasing doses may result in respiratory depression. May also cause hypotension, especially if given in combination with diazepam. Neurological depression may last several days.

Critical issues: Be ready to intubate after repeated boluses of phenobarbitone if the seizures are unremitting.

Phenytoin

Reduces neuronal excitability by acting on the sodium channels.

Onset of action: Peak effect occurs in 15–20 minutes.

Dose: Loading dose is 15–20 mg/kg, given at a rate no faster than 0·5 mg/kg/min.

Side effects: Bradycardia, cardiac arrhythmias, and hypotension.

Critical issues: Due to side effects, must be given under cardiovascular monitoring. Phenytoin precipitates in dextrose solution therefore must be given in saline. It is also an antiarrhythmic agent.

Phenytoin is useful in the head injured patient as it does not cause sedation.

Some neurosurgeons recommend prophylactic phenytoin in paralysed children following serious head injuries.

Not widely used in neonatal intensive care.

Paraldehyde

Although it is one of the oldest, it is also one of the most effective anticonvulsants. Most commonly given per rectally.

Dose: 0·3 ml/kg, plus 0·3 ml/kg arachis oil.

Side effects: Can cause corrosion of rectal mucosa, or a skin rash or hepatitis.

Critical issues: Dissolves PVC, therefore polypropylene syringes should be used. Use with caution in patients with respiratory disease as it is mainly excreted by the lungs.

Clonazepam

Increasingly used to control neonatal seizures resistant to phenobarbitone.

Dose: 50–100 micrograms/kg, maximum 1 mg, as slow IV bolus over 30 minutes once daily, for a maximum of three doses. An infusion of 10–30 micrograms/kg/h may be started after the first dose if seizure control is difficult.

Side effects: Respiratory depression, hypotonia, and increased upper airway and salivary secretions. Side effects may be severe, requiring ventilation, and may interfere with neurological assessment.

Midazolam

Relatively new addition to anticonvulsant regimen. Relatively safe when used as an infusion on its own up to fairly high doses. Minimal respiratory depression.

Antiarrhythmics

Clinical evidence of compromise should be sought before embarking on treatment. See chapter 9. Consultation with a paediatric cardiologist is recommended if at all possible before giving antiarrhythmics.

Consideration must be given to electrically converting abnormal rhythms in appropriate clinical circumstances.

Antiarrhythmic agents are classified based on their electrophysiological effects.

Class I: these drugs block sodium channels, thereby reducing the excitability of the heart.
Class II: these drugs act by beta-adrenoceptor antagonism.
Class III: act by prolonging the refractory period of the myocardium, suppressing re-entrant rhythms.
Class IV: these drugs are Ca^{2+} channel antagonists that impair impulse propagation in nodal areas of the heart.

Supraventricular tachycardia

This can be treated with the drugs described below.

Adenosine

The drug used most commonly if vagal manoeuvres have not succeeded in stopping the arrhythmia. It slows conduction across the AV node.

Dose: With continuous cardiovascular monitoring, the drug is given as a rapid intravenous bolus of 0·05 mg/kg. If there is no effect, the dose may be doubled. The maximum dose is 12 mg. As adenosine has a very short half-life, it should be administered rapidly and immediately followed with a bolus of saline.

Side effects: Bradycardia, hypotension, and flushing.

Critical issues: It is very short acting, i.e. 10 seconds, and its side effects are transient. Must be administered as a rapid push, followed by a rapid saline bolus. It may not work well if the child is acidotic. More effective if given centrally.

Digoxin

Its major drawback in acute supraventricular tachycardia is that conversion takes some time.

Dose: 20–30 micrograms/kg, half of the loading dose initially followed by a quarter in two divided doses at 8–12 hour intervals.

Side effects: Bradycardia, AV block, bigeminy, and trigeminy. Nausea and vomiting, hyperkalaemia, and visual disturbances.

Critical issues: Electrolytes must be normal when on digoxin treatment.

Flecainide

A type 1 antiarrhythmic agent generally used as a second line agent in those patients unresponsive to conventional therapy.

Dose: Starting with 1–2 mg/kg, building up to 3–6 mg/kg/day in three divided doses.

Side effects: Can cause bradycardia and heart block.

Critical issues: Interacts with various drugs including digoxin, amiodarone, and beta-blockers.

Amiodarone

Class III antiarrhythmic agent which is used in the management of resistant life threatening ventricular arrhythmias or unresponsive supraventricular tachycardias.

Onset of action: Even when given intravenously can be a few hours.

Dose: 5 mg/kg over 30–60 minutes. Maintenance dose when used as a continuous infusion is 7–15 mg/kg/day.

Side effects: Potentially numerous. Can cause bradyarrhythmias, second and third degree AV block, discolouration of the skin, and hypothyroidism.

Critical issues: Amiodarone is light sensitive and should be administered via a central line.
   Watch for its negative inotropic effect.

Ventricular arrhythmias

These are most commonly treated with amiodarone or cardioversion, but in resistant cases the following may be considered.

Lidocaine (lignocaine)

Class I antiarrhythmic agent useful for ventricular arrhythmias, and clinically significant premature ventricular contractions.

Onset of action: 45–90 seconds.

Dose: Loading dose of 1 mg/kg/dose. Infusion can be given at 10–50 micrograms/kg/min.

Side effects: Bradycardia, hypotension, and heart block.

Critical issues: Can be given via the endotracheal tube in the same dose.

Antihypertensives

Beta-adrenergic blockers are antihypertensive and antiarrhythmic agents. They act by a number of mechanisms:

- A reduction of renin release from the kidney
- A reduction in cardiac output
- A reduction of sympathetic activity via a central action.

Propranolol

A non-selective beta-blocker.

Onset of action: 20–30 minutes.

Dose: 0·05–0·1 mg/kg.

Side effects: Bronchoconstriction, hypoglycaemia, and cardiac failure.

Critical issues: Is also used in treating cyanotic spells in tetralogy of Fallot.

Labetalol

Blocks both alpha- and beta-receptors.

Onset of action: 2–5 minutes.

Dose: 0·2–1 mg/kg, followed by an IV infusion of 0·25–1·5 mg/kg/h.

Side effects: Similar to propanolol.

Critical issues: Useful for hypertensive emergencies.

Nifedipine

A calcium channel blocker that prevents the influx of Ca^{2+} through the cell membrane and therefore blocks contraction of smooth muscle. The ensuing vasodilatation causes a fall in blood pressure.

Onset of action: 2–5 minutes when administered sublingually, 20 minutes when given orally.

Dose: 0·2–0·5 mg/kg/dose for hypertensive emergencies. Maximum 1–2 mg/kg/day, oral or sublingual.

Side effects: Hypotension, syncope, and dizziness. Hyperglycaemia and hyperuricaemia.

Hydralazine

Produces a drop in blood pressure by causing vasodilatation of arteries and arterioles.

Onset of action: 5–20 minutes.

Dose: 0·1–0·2 mg/kg/dose every 6 hours up to a maximum of 3·5 mg/kg/day.

Side effects: Hypotension, tachycardia.

Critical issues: Hypotension will usually respond to IV fluids or Trendelenburg positioning.

Sodium nitroprusside

Another potent arterial vasodilator. Useful drug for a hypertensive crisis.

Onset of action: Within 2 minutes.

Dose: 0·5–5 micrograms/kg/min.

Side effects: Hypotension and the possibility of cyanide toxicity when used for long periods of time.

Critical issues: Can only be administered as a continuous infusion.

Should be protected from light. Watch for acidosis as a possible indication of cyanide toxicity.

Must not be used to treat hypertension related to increased intracranial pressure due to loss of cerebral autoregulation and the risk of further increasing intracranial pressure.

Neonatal respiratory drugs

Surfactant

Reduces the pulmonary problems associated with surfactant-deficient respiratory distress in preterm babies in the first three days of life. Two surfactant preparations are widely used in the UK—poractant (Curosurf) and beractant (Survanta). Treatment protocols that are prophylactic and rescue oriented are variously followed. Intubated newborn premature babies who have an oxygen requirement over 30% and a chest radiograph consistent with hyaline membrane disease should have surfactant prior to transfer. If a baby needs intubating for transfer then surfactant should be given.

Dose:

Curosurf: 200 mg/kg (2·5 ml/kg) single bolus into trachea. Two further doses of half this amount can be given at 12 hourly intervals.

Survanta: 100 mg/kg (4 ml/kg) bolus into trachea. Two further doses of this amount can be given at 8–12 hour intervals.

Side effects: Transient episodes of bradycardia, decreased oxygen saturation, reflux of the surfactant into the endotracheal tube, and airway obstruction have occurred during dosing with surfactant. These events require interrupting the administration of surfactant and taking the appropriate measures to alleviate the condition. After stabilisation, dosing may resume with appropriate monitoring.

Critical issues: Surfactant can produce rapid improvements in lung compliance and oxygenation that may require immediate reductions in ventilator settings and inspired oxygen. Administration of surfactant should never be less than 30 minutes prior to departure on transport, and blood gases and ventilator settings must be reassessed following surfactant administration prior to undertaking transfer.

Fluids

Administration of fluids intravenously is usually one of the first steps in resuscitating critically ill patients. Crystalloids, plasma, albumin or synthetic colloids such as gelatin, dextran and hydroxyethyl starches are current options for this purpose.

Intravenous fluid administration is well tolerated if the microvascular integrity is preserved but the inflammatory response that occurs in sepsis, trauma, shock and anaphylaxis results in increased intravascular permeability.

Significant vascular leakage causes interstitial oedema which may adversely affect organ function: cerebral oedema causes mental status changes, pulmonary oedema impairs gas exchange, myocardial oedema decreases compliance and impairs myocardial function.

It is still not clear whether crystalloids or colloids are better for resuscitation. Suffice to say, whichever (crystalloid or colloid) is readily available in an acute emergency should be used.

For ongoing resuscitation, colloids would be the appropriate solutions to use because although there is no evidence to suggest colloids are better than crystalloids, there is some evidence to support the view that colloids resuscitate the circulation more efficiently and cause less oedema due to leakage from the intravascular space.

Crystalloid

The crystalloids used most commonly are isotonic saline and Ringer's lactate. Both are confined to the extracellular space due to the sodium content. A high proportion ends up in the interstitial space, contributing to interstitial oedema.

A possible advantage of Ringer's lactate is that it contains lactate which is converted into base by a functioning liver and may additionally biochemically help the pH. Studies are underway looking at the use of hypertonic saline following head injuries and for resuscitation following major trauma.

Colloid

Colloids have an oncotic pressure that is provided by large molecules similar in size to human albumin. Albumin (4·5% human albumin solution) has a molecular weight of 69 000 daltons and lasts in the circulation for about 3–4 hours. It is derived from pooled human serum and therefore has the potential risk of infecting the recipient. It is also expensive.

Gelofusine is a gelatine with a molecular weight of 35 000 daltons and lasts in the circulation for about 2–3 hours, less time than other artificial colloids.

Pentastarch is a polymerised carbohydrate with a molecular weight of 450 000 daltons and lasts in the circulation for about 4–6 hours. It is thought to have many attractive properties such as a reduction of oedema in inflammatory states and an improvement of microcirculatory flow.

How much to administer?

Newborn infants: Start with 10 ml/kg. This group rarely require more than 20 ml/kg of volume replacement, unless there is clear evidence of blood or fluid loss. Anticipate the need for volume replacement when transferring infants with gastroschisis or who have a perforated bowel. Use blood transfusion if blood loss is the problem or the patient is anaemic.

Older children: In the acutely hypovolaemic child, it may be necessary to administer 20 ml/kg as a bolus in the first instance. This must then be followed up by constant evaluation.

This bolus can be repeated if signs of hypovolaemia persist. Consideration should be given to monitoring the central venous pressure if the child needs more than 40 ml/kg fluid resuscitation.

A child with hypovolaemic shock may often require 40–60 ml/kg of fluid in the first hour. Large fluid requirements in septic shock should also make one consider the need to support ventilation.

Depending on the clinical situation, fluid replacement with blood should be considered after about 40 ml/kg of fluid has been given.

Drug prescription and administration

Transported infants and children should have all drugs prescribed, checked and administered to the same high standard that they would receive on the intensive care unit. The transport record should clearly show what drugs were given, in what doses, when and who prescribed, checked and administered them. It is sometimes necessary on transport for the person prescribing a drug to also be involved in checking and administering, simply because there are fewer pairs of hands. Try to avoid this if possible, for example by recruiting the help of the local team, as there is increased potential for prescription errors to be duplicated in the checking process.

Prescription errors are more likely under pressure or in a crisis. One activity the transport team can attend to on the way to a retrieval, presuming they are not prone to motion sickness, is precalculation and checking of doses for drugs that may be needed, based on the weight of the infant or child given at referral.

In general the transport team should reserve any drugs carried in transport packs, and use local unit supplies wherever possible, to avoid depleting supplies that may be needed on the return journey.

Advanced neonatal nurse practitioners (ANNPs) who lead transfers will need to undertake the prescribing-like activity provided for under the Patient Group Directives (PGD) framework. Local unit and hospital policy will determine the precise structure and contents of PGDs. Drugs initiated by ANNPs should be regularly and rigorously audited to ensure that both the letter and spirit of the supporting documents are being followed. Nurse prescribing in general is a rapidly evolving area, and future developments may more overtly facilitate prescribing for nurses in intensive care.

Appendix 1: Typical retrieval forms

Samples of transport documentation used by paediatric and neonatal transport teams are reproduced over the next pages.

Documentation will inevitably be tailored to suit the operational protocols and characteristics of individual teams. There are some important principles underpinning these documents which should apply to all transport documentation.

A proper record should be made and kept of every transfer. This has a number of purposes. Firstly, the receiving team will need a good record of the care and treatment the patient has received. Secondly, the form may act as an aide-mémoire, reminding you of routine procedures that need attending to. Finally, this is your defence in cases where negligence is alleged and where there will otherwise be an undocumented gap in the care record. It will not be enough merely to assert that as there were two people on the transfer with a sick child, it stands to reason you must have been observing and caring for the child in a competent manner. Remember that by the time the conduct of the transfer is legally challenged all concerned may well have no memory of it. The documentation should include information that will allow reconstruction of the key features of the transfer—who attended, times, clinical findings and interventions, drugs used, and observations taken.

During the actual journey, record observations and fluids more frequently than on the unit— every 15–30 minutes. This recognises the additional hazards of transfer over unit work. An entry should be made in the patient's medical notes about both the stabilisation and transfer.

Once a good record has been made, it is important that it is kept. Discuss the forms with the medical records department to ensure they appreciate their importance, and that they are properly filed. Duplicate forms are useful, where one copy goes in the notes and another is held by the transport office.

NOTTINGHAM NEONATAL SERVICE TRANSPORT RECORD (1)   DATE

A.GIBBS.01/00

NAME

DATE OF BIRTH	NAME BANDS	E.T.T. SIZE
REFERRAL HOSPITAL	TIME OF BIRTH	CUT AT
REFERRAL HOSPITAL NO.	AGE	LAST TUBE CHANGE DATE
MOTHERS TRANSFER PLAN	CONTACT NO.	GUTHRIE/TSH

Time																							
P.I.P																							
P.E.E.P./C.P.A.P.																							
Ti. Time																							
Ventilator Rate																							
Respiratory Rate																							
FiO_2																							
Saturation																							
$TcPO_2$																							
$TcPCO_2$																							
E.T.T. Washout/Suction																							
Heart Rate																							
Bp Mean																							
Systolic/Diastolic																							
Baby Temperature																							
Incubator Temperature																							
Comments/Actions Location																							

NAME	SIGNATURE

NOTTINGHAM NEONATAL SERVICE TRANSPORT RECORD (2)   DATE

A.GIBBS.01/00

NAME   D.O.B.   HOSP NO.   DRUGS

BIRTH WT.   PRESENT WT.   Vit K. O/I.M.

Time	fluids mls/kg	ml/hr	Total	site	ml/hr	Total	site	ml/hr	Total	site	ml/hr	Total	site	ml/hr	Total	site	ml/hr	Total	site	blood sugar	NG ASP		Urine	Bowels	

HISTORY

STABILISATION

IN TRANSIT

NAME   SIGNATURE

Nottingham Neonatal Emergency Transport Service – Audit Form

Baby:

Name:	CHN number:	Birth weight:
	QMC number:	Weight at transfer:
Date:	D.O.B:	Gestation at birth:	Age at transfer:

Baby moved from: **Baby moved to:**

Unit:	Hospital:	Unit:	Hospital

Journey:

1. Referral accepted:	2. Vehicle requested:	3. Vehicle arrived:	4. Vehicle mobile:
5. Arrival at referring unit::	6. Departure:	7. Arrival at destination:	

Further times:

Baby attended by team but not transferred:	Baby died in transit:	

Please explain any delays apparent from the times given:

Personnel/Family/Diagnosis:

Transport Nurse:	Doctor/ANNP:	Grade of doctor:

Learner(s) (Name and type of learner):

Mother seen? Y/N	Father seen? Y/N	Video seen? Y/N	Babyfax given? Y/N

Diagnosis:	Reason for transfer:

Appropriate?   Y/N

Procedures:

Which of these was performed, attempted or initiated by the transport team?

1st Intubation:	Extubation:	Reintubation:	Surfactant:	UAC:
Peripheral art.line:	UVC:	Chest needled:	Blood culture:	Antibotics:
Sedation:	Muscle relaxation:	Inotropes:	CPR:	ETT Suction (n=):
Blood gas (n=):	X-Ray (n=):	Chest drains (n=):	IV Cannula (n=):	

Transport Score:

Please complete **score one** on arrival at the referring unit, before you intervene. If possible, do a **second score** before departure to reflect how the stabilising period has gone. **Score three** should be completed when the baby is settled in a static incubator at the end of the journey. If only capillary pO_2 is available, record the TINA and saturation readings

	0	1	2
1. Blood Glucose	< 1·3	1·3–2·2 or > 9·7	2·3–9·7
2. Systolic Blood Pressure	< 30	30–40	> 40
3. pH	< 7·2 or >7·5	7·2–7·29 or 7·46–7·5	7·3–7·45
4. pO_2	< 5·3	5·3–6·5 or > 13	6·6–13
5. Temperature	< 36·1 or >37·6	36·1–36·5 or 37·3–37·6	36·6–37·2

Score one:	1/	2/	3/	4/	5/	TOTAL:
Actual values:	1/	2/	3/	4/	5/	

Score two:	1/	2/	3/	4/	5/	TOTAL:
Actual values:	1/	2/	3/	4/	5/	

Score three:	1/	2/	3/	4/	5/	TOTAL:
Actual values:	1/	2/	3/	4/	5/	

AJL 0100

In Transit

Equipment & monitoring:
Tick any of these items used during transfer

ECG:	Ventilator:	INCA CPAP:	Prong CPAP/IMV:	Humid-vent:
Oxygen:	Pulse-oximeter:	Arterial BP:	Dinamap BP:	O_2 analyser:
Temp. probe:	SureTemp:	TINA (no ABG cal):	TINA (pO_2 cal):	TINA (pCO_2 cal):
Vehicle call-code:		Graseby pump:	System 1 or 2:	Nitric Oxide:

I.V. and I.A. fluids and drugs required in transit. Please tick:

Maintenance fluids		Other infusions			
10% Glucose	10% Glucose and 0·18% Saline	Heparinised Saline	Diamorphine	Midazolam	Sodium bicarbonate
15% Glucose	4% Glucose and 0·18% Saline	0·9% Saline	Dobutamine	Morphine	Tolazoline
5% Glucose		Albumin 4·5%	Dopamine	Pancuronium	
Other:		Atracurium	Epinephrine 1:10,000	Prostacyclin	
		Blood	Magnesium Sulphate	Prostaglandin	
		Other:			

Respiratory support:

Start of journey:	Mode:	PIP:	PEEP/CPAP:	BPM:	FiO_2:
End of journey:	Mode:	PIP:	PEEP/CPAP:	BPM:	FiO_2:
Maximum settings:	Mode:	PIP:	PEEP/CPAP:	BPM:	FiO_2:

Problems:

Did any equipment fail, or give problems?

Were there any problems with the baby in transit?

Action taken:

Please phone other units for final scores if necessary

IMPORTANT: Check this form is complete before filing – a mark in every box

AJL 0100

PAEDIATRIC INTENSIVE CARE – LEICESTER
RETRIEVAL DOCUMENTATION

Important: Fill in this document as completely and legibly as possible!
TELEPHONE CALL

Call received by   **Name:** _____

Date: _____ / _____ / _____   **Time:** _____

Reason for contact: [Transfer]   [Advice only]

Referring doctor and grade: _____   **Bleep no:** _____

Referring consultant: _____   **Aware:**   [Yes] [No]

Referring hospital: _____

Date of admission to referring hospital: _____ / _____ / _____   **Time:** _____

Location of patient: [A&E][ITU][NNU][PICU][Other _____]

Hospital telephone number: _____   **Extension:** _____

PATIENT DATA

Name: _____   **Sex:** [M][F]

D.O.B: _____   **Age:** _____   **Weight:** _____ Kg

Provisional diagnosis: _____

Brief history including premorbid conditions:

_____

_____

_____

_____

_____

_____

_____

_____

CURRENT STATUS AT REFERRING HOSPITAL

Intubated   [Yes] [No]

If intubated:	Time: _____

Ventilated: [Yes][No][Handbagged]

  Ventilator: _____

ETT: size _____ length _____ [O][N]

Rate _____ /min TV _____ ml MV _____ L

PIP _____ cmH$_2$O   PEEP _____ cmH$_2$O

OI[FiO$_2$(%)xMAP/PaO$_2$(mmHg)] _____

NO (ppm) _____

CXR _____

%SaO$_2$ _____ in _____ FiO$_2$

If not intubated:

Resp rate: _____ /min

Resp distress: [None][Mid]

                    [Moderate][Severe]

Stridor: [Y][N]   Wheeze: [Y][N]

Added sounds: _____

Air entry: [Normal][Abnormal]

              [R=L][R>L][R<L]

CXR: _____

%SaO$_2$ _____ in _____ FiO$_2$

Pulse: _____ /min   **BP:** _____/_____ mmHg   **Capillary refill:** _____ seconds

Colour: [Pink] [Pale] [Cyanosed]   **Temperature: Core:** _____ **Peripheral:** _____ °C

Heart sounds: [Normal] [Abnormal]   **Gallop:** [Yes] [No]   **Murmur:** [Yes] [No]

Liver: _____ cms   **Spleen:** _____ cms   **Urine output:** _____ ml/kg/hour

Level of consciousness:

  [Alert]   **Pupils:**   **Right:** _____ mm   [Brisk][Sluggish][Fixed]

  [Responds to voice]   **Left:** _____ mm   [Brisk][Sluggish][Fixed]

  [Responds to pain]   **Fundi:** _____

  [Unresponsiveness]

  [Paralysed and sedated]   **Meningism:**   [Yes] [No]

Rash: _____

MOST RECENT BLOOD RESULTS

Biochemistry	Result	Blood Gas	Result
Glucose		pH	
Sodium		PCO$_2$	
Potassium		pO$_2$/FiO$_2$	/
Urea		Bicarbonate	
Creatinine		Base deficit	
Calcium		**Haematology**	
Bilirubin		Hb	
Albumin		WCC	
		Platelets	
		INR	
		APTT	

TREATMENT ALREADY GIVEN BY REFERRING HOSPITAL

Lines: Peripheral venous lines: _____

Central venous line: [Yes] [No] [Site _____] Arterial lines: [Yes] [No]

Fluids given: Colloid _____ ml/kg   FFP _____ ml/kg

Blood _____ ml/kg   Other _____ ml/kg

Inotropes/   Name _____ rate _____ mcg/kg/min

Vasodilators   Name _____ rate _____ mcg/kg/min

Name _____ rate _____ mcg/kg/min

Maintenance fluid   Type _____ rate _____ ml/kg/day = _____ ml/hr

[Normal] [Restrict to _____ %] [Increase to _____ %]

Drugs given   **(Name, dose, time)** _____

_____

_____

CHECKLIST WITH REFERRING DOCTOR

If accepted for transfer ask for the following to be done before Retrieval Team arrives

[   ]   TWO IV lines needed

[   ]   Stop oral or NG feeding, insert NGT if intubating

[   ]   Notify parents of transfer

[   ]   Photocopy A&E, medical and nursing notes/obs and copy/borrow Xrays

Additional requests for **ECMO patients:**

[   ]   Full clotting screen

[   ]   Head scan (and heart scan if possible)

[   ]   Cross match for blood: 10ml clotted sample from mother (if neonate)

1 adult unit (300ml) of packed cells

TRANSFER TEAM DETAILS

Nurses: 1. _____   2. _____

Doctors: 1. _____   2. _____

TRANSFER TIMES

Time ambulance booked: _____

Time of departure from Leicester: _____

Time of arrival at referring hospital: _____

Time of departure from referring hospital: _____

Time of arrival at Leicester: _____

CONDITION ON ARRIVAL OF RETRIEVAL TEAM
(Assessment by Medical Team)

Intubated   [Yes] [No]

If intubated: Time: _____	**If not intubated:**
Ventilated: [Yes][No][Handbagged]	Resp rate: _____ /min
Ventilator: _____	Resp distress: [None][Mid]
ETT: size _____ length _____ [O][N]	[Moderate][Severe]
Rate _____/min TV _____ml MV _____ L	Stridor: [Y] [N] Wheeze: [Y] [N]
PIP _____ cmH$_2$O PEEP _____ cmH$_2$O	Added sounds: _____
OI[FiO$_2$(%)xMAP/PaO$_2$(mmHg)] _____	Air entry: [Normal][Abnormal]
NO (ppm) _____	[R=L][R>L][R<L]
CXR _____	CXR: _____
%SaO$_2$ _____ in _____ FiO$_2$	%SaO$_2$ _____ in _____ FiO$_2$

Pulse: _____ /min   **BP:** _____ mmHg   **Capillary refill:** _____ seconds

Colour: [Pink] [Pale] [Cyanosed]   **Temperature: Core:** _____ **Peripheral:** _____ °C

Heart sounds: [Normal] [Abnormal]   **Gallop:** [Yes] [No]   **Murmur:** [Yes] [No]

Liver: _____ cms   **Spleen:** _____ cms   **Urine output:** _____ ml/kg/hour

Level of consciousness:

   [Alert]   **Pupils:**   **Right:** _____ mm   [Brisk][Sluggish][Fixed]

   [Responds to voice]   **Left:** _____ mm   [Brisk][Sluggish][Fixed]

   [Responds to pain]   **Fundi:** _____

   [Unresponsiveness]

   [Paralysed and sedated]   **Meningism:**   [Yes] [No]

Other findings: _____

_____

_____

_____

_____

_____

_____

Dactors name: _____   **Signature:** _____

ACTIONS TAKEN BY TRANSFER TEAM

Airway: Intubated/Tube changed   [Yes][No]   Time: _____

ETT: Size: _____ Length: _____   [Oral] [Nasal]

Drugs used for intubation: _____

Ventilator   FiO$_2$: _____   PIP: _____   PEEP: _____

settings: Rate: _____   Ti : _____   Te: _____

Access: Peripheral cannulae   exiting: _____   put in by TT: _____

Central venous line: exiting: _____   put in by TT: _____

Arterial line: exiting: _____   put in by TT: _____

Urinary catheter: [Present] [Passed] [Changed] [None]

NG tube: [Present] [Passed] [Changed] [None]

Antibiotics: _____   Time: _____

Other treatments: _____

_____

_____

_____

_____

PRE-DEPARTURE CHECKLIST

CLINICAL STATUS
Airway	Airway secure, ETT securely fixed	[	]
Ventilation	Ventilation satisfactory, Blood gases, Chest Xray	[	]
Circulation	Adequate fluids/inotropes, Vascular access secure	[	]
Neurology	Seizures controlled, Adequately sedated/paralysed	[	]
Renal	Urinary catheter in place if required	[	]
GIT	NG tube passed if required, blood sugar satisfactory	[	]
Temperature	Measured and satisfactory, Adequate warming	[	]

DOCUMENTATION   [Notes]   [Letter]   [Transfer consent]   [Xrays]

SUPPLIES   [Oxygen]   [Fluids]   [Power]

COMMUNICATION   [Parents][Parent package given]

ON TROLLEY   [Mask]   [Resus drugs]   [Rebreathe bag]   [Stethoscope]

BAGS   [Drugs box][Fridge drugs]   [Red/Green bag]

TELEPHONE   [PICU Leicester notified]

ECMO PATIENTS   [Blood]   [ECMO Consent]

Nursing evaluation and notes during transfer: _____

_____

_____

_____

_____

_____

_____

_____

_____

_____

_____

_____

_____

_____

_____

Nurses name and grade: _____   **Signature:** _____

CONDITION ON ARRIVAL BACK IN LEICESTER

Temperature: Core: _____ °C   Peripheral: _____ °C

Ventilation FiO_2: _____   PIP: _____   PEEP: _____

                         Rate: _____   Ti : _____   Te: _____

                         SpO_2 _____ $etCO_2$ _____

Haemodynamics: Pulse: _____   BP: _____   Cap refill: _____

Neurology: GCS: _____   Pupils: _____

UNTOWARD EVENTS

PATIENT   EQUIPMENT

Awake	[ ]	Desaturation	[ ]	Ventilator failure	[ ]	Monitor failure	[ ]
Hypotension	[ ]	Rise in $etCO_2$	[ ]	Inf. pump failure	[ ]	Loss of IV	[ ]
Hypertension	[ ]	Extubation	[ ]	Failed gas supply	[ ]	Communication	[ ]
Bradycardia	[ ]	ETT blocked	[ ]	Ambulance prob	[ ]		
Tachycardia	[ ]	Pupil changes	[ ]	Bag not equipped	[ ]		
Other	[ ]	Specify: _____					

Brief details of event: _____

_____

Incident form completed   Yes [ ]   No [ ]

Appendix 2: Essential equations and aide-mémoires

Estimating weight

Weight (kg) = (age + 4) × 2

Blood gas unit conversion

To convert mmHg to kPa, multiply by 0·1317.
To convert kPa to mmHg, divide by 0·1317.

Respiratory support indices

Oxygenation index (OI) = mean airway pressure × Fio_2 (%)/Pao_2 in mmHg.

Ventilation index (VI) = $Paco_2$ × respiratory rate × peak inspiratory pressure/1000

Mean airway pressure = ((PIP × T_I) + (PEEP × T_e))/ (T_I + T_e)

where PIP = peak inspiratory pressure
PEEP = positive end expiratory pressure
T_I = inspiratory time
T_e = expiratory time

Other physiological measures

Oxygen content in blood = 1·36 × Hb × oxygen saturation

Desired systolic blood pressure = 80 + (age × 2) (over 2 years of age)

Anion gap = (Na^+ + K^+) − (CL^- + HCO_3^-)

Osmolality (serum) = (2 × Na^+) + glucose + urea

Gas requirements for transfer

The oxygen requirements (in litres) of a patient can be estimated from the formula:

Flow delivered (l/min) × Fio_2 × journey time (min) × 2

How long a cylinder supply will last may be estimated from the formula:

Cylinder contents (litres)/gas consumption (litres/min)

(approximate cylinder contents when full are printed on the cylinder)

Endotracheal tube sizes

Rough guide for infant ETT internal diameter – gestation/10 (also see table below). Older child ETT sizes:
Diameter: (age/4) + 4
Length (oral ETT): (age/2) + 12
Length (nasal ETT): (age/4) + 15

Weight (g)	ETT diameter	Oral endotracheal tubes Cut length	Length at lips	Nasal tubes Length at nares
500	2·5	6·5	6	7·5
1000	2·5	7	6·5	8·5
1500	2·5–3·0	7·5	7	9
2000	3·0	8	7·5	9·5
2500	3·0	8·5	8	10
3000	3·5	9·5	9	10·5
3500	3·5	10·5	10	11·5

Selected references and bibliography

General

Advanced Life Support Group. *Advanced Paediatric Life Support*. London: BMJ Publishing Group, 1997.

Advanced Life Support Group. *Safe Transfer and Retrieval—The Practical Approach*. London: BMJ Publishing Group, 2002.

Booth P, Madar J, Skeoch C. *The Handbook of Neonatal Transport*. Aberdeen: Scottish Neonatal Consultants' Group, 1996.

British Paediatric Association. *The Care of Critically Ill Children*. Report of a Multidisciplinary Working Party on Paediatric Intensive Care. London: British Paediatric Association, 1993.

Glasgow JFT, Graham HK. *Management of Injuries in Children*. London: BMJ Publishing Group, 1997.

Jaimovich DG, Vidyasagar D (eds). *Handbook of Pediatric and Neonatal Transport Medicine*. Philadelphia: Hanley and Belfus, 1996.

Macnab AJ, Smart P. Lightweight monitoring equipment for pediatric transport. *Intens Ther Clin Monit* 1990;(May/June):92–6.

Macrae DJ. Paediatric intensive care transport. *Arch Dis Child* 1994;**71**:175–8.

Morton NS, Pollack MM, Wallace PGM (eds). *Stabilisation and Transport of the Critically Ill*. Edinburgh: Churchill Livingstone, 1997.

Resuscitation Council (UK). *Newborn Life Support Provider Course Manual*. London: Resuscitation Council, 2001.

Resuscitation Council (UK). *Resuscitation Guidelines 2000*. London: Resuscitation Council, 2000.

Principles of safe transport

Anonymous. Guidelines for the transfer of critically ill patients. *Crit Care Med* 1993;**21**:931–7.

Barry PW, Ralston C. Adverse events occurring during interhospital transfer of the critically ill. *Arch Dis Child* 1994;**71**:8–11.

Britto J, Nadel S, Levin M, Habibi P. Mobile paediatric intensive care: the ethos of transferring critically ill children. *Care Crit Ill* 1995;**11**:235–8.

Edge WE, Kanter RK, Weigle CGM, Walsh RF. Reduction in morbidity in inter-hospital transport by specialized pediatric staff. *Crit Care Med* 1994;**22**:1186–91.

Intensive Care Society. *Guidelines for the Transport of the Critically Ill Adult*. London: Intensive Care Society, 1997.

Hunt RC, Brown LH, Cabinum ES, et al. Is ambulance transport time with lights and sirens faster than that without? *Ann Emerg Med* 1995;**25**:507–11.

Leslie A, Bose C. Nurse-led neonatal transport. *Semin Neonatol* 1999;**4**:265–71.

Logan S. Evaluation of specialist paediatric retrieval teams. *Br Med J* 1995;**311**:839.

Lovell MA, Mudaliar MY, Klineberg PL. Intrahospital transport of critically ill patients: complications and difficulties. *Anaesth Intens Care* 2001;**29**:400–5.

Macnab AJ. Optimal escort for inter-hospital transport of pediatric emergencies. *J Trauma* 1991;**31**:205–9.

Macrae DJ. Paediatric intensive care transport. *Arch Dis Child* 1994;**71**:175–8.

Paediatric Intensive Care Society. *Standards for Paediatric Intensive Care Including Standards of Practice for the Transportation of the Critically Ill Child*. Paediatric Intensive Care Society, 1996: Bishop's Stortford, UK: Saldatore.

Pon S, Notterman DA. The organisation of a pediatric critical care transport program. *Pediatr Clin North Am* 1993;**40**:241–61.

Sharples PM. Avoidable factors contributing to death of children with head injury. *Br Med J* 1990;**300**:87–91.

Transport physiology

Gajendragadkar G, Boyd JA, Potter DW, Mellen BG, Hahn GD, Shenai JP. Mechanical vibration in neonatal transport: a randomized study of different mattresses. *J Perinatol* 2000;**20**:307–10.

Lawler PG. Transfer of critically ill patients: Part 1—physiological concepts. *Care Crit Ill* 2000;**16**:61–5.

Lawler PG. Transfer of critically ill patients: Part 2—preparation for transfer. *Care Crit Ill* 2000;**16**:94–7.

Miller C. The physiologic effects of air transport on the neonate. *Neonatal Network* 1994;**13**:7–10.

Sherwood HB, Donze A, Giebe J. Mechanical vibration in ambulance transport. *Clin Studies* 1994;**23**:457–63.

Towers CV, Bonebrake R, Padilla G, Rumney P. The effect of transport on the rate of severe intraventricular hemorrhage in very low birth weight infants. *Obstet Gynecol* 2000;**95**:291–5.

Wright MS, Bose CL, Stiles AD. The incidence and effects of motion sickness among medical attendants during transport. *J Emerg Med* 1995;**13**:15–20.

The ambulance environment

Auerbach P, Morris J, Phillips J, et al. An analysis of ambulance accidents in Tennessee. *JAMA* 1987;**258**:487–90.

Lacher ME, Bausher JC. Lights and siren in pediatric 911 ambulance transports: are they being misused? *Ann Emerg Med* 1997;**29**:223–7.

Little JW. Ambulance transport for the newborn. *Semin Neonatol* 1999;**4**:247–51.

Madar RJ, Milligan DWA. Neonatal transport: safety and security. *Arch Dis Child* 1994;**71**:F147–8.

Medical Devices Agency. *Transport of Neonates in Ambulances (TINA)*. London: Department of Health, 1995.

Equipment and monitoring

Brown L, Gough JE, Bryan-Berg D, Hunt R. Assessment of breath sounds during ambulance transport. *Ann Emerg Med* 1997;**29**:228–31.

Gebremichael M, Borg U, Habashi NM, et al. Interhospital transport of the extremely ill patient: the mobile intensive care unit. *Crit Care Med* 2000;**28**:79–85.

Palmon SC, Liu M, Moore LE, Kirsch JR. Capnography facilitates tight control of ventilation during transport. *Crit Care Med* 1996;**24**:608–11.

Wilson C, Webber S. Oxygenation saturation during transfer. *Paediatr Anaesth* 2002;**12**:288.

Air transport of critically ill children

Aoki BY, McCloskey K. *Evaluation, Stabilisation and Transport of the Critically Ill Child*. St Louis: Mosby Year Book, 1992.

Bjerke HS, Barcliff L, Foglia RP. Neonatal survival during a 2500-mile flight. *Hawaii Med J* 1992;**51**:332–5.

Neonatal resuscitation and stabilisation

Utility of trained teams

Chance G, Matthew J, Gash J, et al. Neonatal transport: a controlled study of skilled assistance. *J Pediatr* 1978;**93**:662–6.

Cook L, Kattwinkel J. A prospective study of nurse-supervised versus physician-supervised neonatal transports. *J Obstet Gynecol Neonatal Nurs* 1983;**12**:371–6.

Hood J, Cross A, Hulka B, et al. Effectiveness of the neonatal transport team. *Crit Care Med* 1983;**11**:419–23.

Leslie A, Bose C. Nurse-led neonatal transport. *Semin Neonatol* 1999;**4**:265–71.

Leslie A, Stephenson T. Audit of neonatal intensive care transport. *Arch Dis Child* 1994;**71**:F61–6.

Leslie A, Stephenson T. Audit of neonatal intensive care transport—closing the loop. *Acta Paediatr* 1997;**86**:1253–6.

Leslie A, Stephenson T. Neonatal transfers by advanced neonatal nurse practitioners and paediatric registrars. *Arch Dis Child* 2003 (in press).

Equipment and monitoring

Nielson H, Jung A, Atherton S. Evaluation of the Porta-Warm Mattress as a source of heat for neonatal transport. *Pediatrics* 1976;**58**:500–4.

O'Connor T, Grueber R. Transcutaneous measurement of carbon dioxide tension during long-distance transport of neonates receiving mechanical ventilation. *J Perinatol* 1998;**18**:189–92.

Vohra S, Frent G, Campbell V, Abbott M, Whyte R. Effect of polyethylene occlusive skin wrapping on heat loss in VLBW infants at delivery: a randomized trial. *J Pediatr* 1999;**134**:547–51.

Others

American Academy of Pediatrics. *Guidelines for Air and Ground Transport of Neonatal and Pediatric Patients*, 2nd edn. Elk Grove, IL: American Academy of Pediatrics, 1999.

Booth P, Madar J, Skeoch C. *The Handbook of Neonatal Transport—A Practical Approach for Scotland*. Aberdeen: Scottish Neonatal Consultants' Group, 1996.

Hellström-Westas L, Hanseus K, Jögi P, Lundström N-R, Svenningsen N. Long-distance transports of newborn infants with congenital heart disease. *Pediatr Cardiol* 2001;**22**:380–4.

Hermansen M, Hasan S, Hoppin J, et al. A validation of a scoring system to evaluate the condition of transported very-low-birth-weight neonates. *Am J Perinatol* 1988;**5**:74–8.

Leslie A, Middleton D. Give and take in neonatal transport: communication hazards in handover. *J Neonatal Nurs* 1995;**1**:27–31.

L'Herault J, Petroff L, Jeffrey J. The effectiveness of a thermal mattress in stabilizing and maintaining body temperature during the transport of very low-birth weight newborns. *Appl Nurs Res* 2001;**14**:210–19.

Medical Devices Agency. *Transport of Neonates in Ambulances (TINA)*. London: Department of Health, 1995.

Stephenson TJ, Marlow N, Watkin S, Grant J. *Pocket Neonatology*. Edinburgh: Churchill Livingstone, 2000.

Management of the airway and breathing

Adams K, Scott R, Perkin RM, Langga L. Comparison of intubation skills between interfacility transport team members. *Pediatr Emerg Care* 2000;**16**(1):5–8.

Dockery WK, Futterman C, Keller SR, Sheridan MJ, Akl BF. A comparison of manual and mechanical ventilation during pediatric transport. *Crit Care Med* 1999;**27**:802–6.

Orf J, Thomas SH, Ahmed W, et al. Appropriateness of endotracheal tube size and insertion depth in children undergoing air medical transport. *Pediatr Emerg Care* 2000;**16**:321–7.

Page NE, Giehl M, Luke S. Intubation complications in the critically ill child. *Adv Pract Acute Crit Care* 1998;**9**:25–35.

Slater EA, Weiss SJ, Ernst AA, Haynes M. Preflight versus en route success and complications of rapid sequence intubation in an air medical service. *J Trauma* 1998;**45**:588–92.

Special transport interventions

Anonymous. Inhaled nitric oxide and hypoxic respiratory failure in infants with congenital diaphragmatic hernia. The Neonatal Inhaled Nitric Oxide Study Group (NINOS). *Pediatrics* 1997;**99**: 838–45.

Anonymous. Inhaled nitric oxide in full-term and nearly full-term infants with hypoxic respiratory failure. The Neonatal Inhaled Nitric Oxide Study Group. *New Engl J Med* 1997;**336**:597–604.

Anonymous. UK collaborative randomised trial of neonatal extracorporeal membrane oxygenation. UK Collaborative ECMO Trial Group. *Lancet* 1996; **348**:75–82.

Baird TM, Paton JB, Fisher DE. Improved oxygenation with prone positioning in neonates: stability of increased transcutaneous Po_2. *J Perinatol* 1991;**11**: 315–18.

Bennett JB, Hill JG, Long WB 3rd, Bruhn PS, Haun MM, Parsons JA. Interhospital transport of the patient on extracorporeal cardiopulmonary support. *Ann Thoracic Surg* 1994;**57**:107–11.

Blythe D. A review of pulmonary vasodilators. *Anaesth Intens Care* 1998;**26**:26–39.

Chang YJ, Anderson GC, Dowling D, Lin CH. Decreased activity and oxygen desaturation in prone ventilated preterm infants during the first postnatal week. *Heart Lung* 2002;**31**:34–42.

Clark RH, Yoder BA, Sell MS. Prospective, randomized comparison of high-frequency oscillation and conventional ventilation in candidates for extracorporeal membrane oxygenation. *J Pediatr* 1994;**124**:447–54.

Cornish JD, Carter JM, Gerstmann DR, Null DM Jr. Extracorporeal membrane oxygenation as a means of stabilizing and transporting high risk neonates. *ASAIO Trans* 1991;**37**:564–8.

Faulkner SC, Taylor BJ, Chipman CW, et al. Mobile extracorporeal membrane oxygenation. *Ann Thor Surg* 1993;**55**:1244–6.

Gattinoni L, Tognoni G, Pesenti A, et al. Effect of prone positioning on the survival of patients with acute respiratory failure. *New Engl J Med* 2001;**345**: 568–73.

Gerstmann DR, Minton SD, Stoddard RA, et al. The Provo multicenter early high-frequency oscillatory ventilation trial: improved pulmonary and clinical outcome in respiratory distress syndrome. *Pediatrics* 1996;**98**:1044–57.

Heulitt MJ, Taylor BJ, Faulkner SC, et al. Inter-hospital transport of neonatal patients on extracorporeal membrane oxygenation: mobile-ECMO. *Pediatrics* 1995;**95**:562–6.

Kinsella JP, Griebel J, Schmidt JM, Abman SH. Use of inhaled nitric oxide during interhospital transport of newborns with hypoxemic respiratory failure. *Pediatrics* 2002;**109**:158–61.

Peek GJ, Firmin RK. Extracorporeal membrane oxygenation for cardiac support. *Coronary Artery Dis* 1997;**8**:371–88.

Peek GJ, Firmin RK. Extracorporeal membrane oxygenation, a favourable outcome? *Br J Anaesth* 1997;**78**:235–7.

Peek GJ, Moore HM, Moore N, Sosnowski AW, Firmin RK. Extracorporeal membrane oxygenation for adult respiratory failure. *Chest* 1997;**112**:759–64.

Peek GJ, Sosnowski AW. Extra-corporeal membrane oxygenation for paediatric respiratory failure. *Br Med Bull* 1997;**53**:745–56.

Ring JC, Stidham GL. Novel therapies for acute respiratory failure. *Pediatr Clin North Am* 1994;**41**: 1325–63.

Roberts JD, Polaner DM, Lang P, Zapol WM. Inhaled nitric oxide in persistent pulmonary hypertension of the newborn. *Lancet* 1992;**340**:818–19.

Shapiro M, Anderson H, Pranikoff T, Chapman R, Bartlett RH. Transport of unstable patients on extracorporeal life support. *Cardiol Young* 1995;(suppl 2):27.

Wagaman MJ, Shutack JG, Moomjian AS, Schwartz JG, Shaffer TH, Fox WW. Improved oxygenation and lung compliance with prone positioning of neonates. *J Pediatr* 1979;**94**:787–91.

What to do when it all goes wrong

Bion JF. Transporting critically ill patients by ambulance: audit by sickness scoring. *Br Med J* 1988;**296**:170.

Britto J, Nadel S, Habibi P, Levin M. Pediatric risk of mortality score underestimates the requirement for intensive care during interhospital transport. *Crit Care Med* 1994;**22**:2029–30.

Britto J, Nadel S, Maconochie I, Levin M, Habibi P. Morbidity and severity of illness during interhospital transfer: impact of specialist paediatric retrieval team. *Br Med J* 1995;**311**:836–9.

Gunnarsson B, Heard CMB, Rotta AT, Heard AMB, Kourkounis BH, Fletcher JE. Use of a physiologic scoring system during interhospital transport of pediatric patients. *Air Med J* 2001;**20**:23–6.

Orr RA, Venkataraman ST, Cinoman MI, Hogue BL, Singleton CA, McCloskey KA. Pretransport pediatric risk of mortality (PRISM) score underestimates the requirement for intensive care or major interventions during interhospital transport. *Crit Care Med* 1994;**22**:101–7.

Woodward GA, Fleegler EW. Should parents accompany pediatric interfacility ground ambulance transports? Results of a national survey of pediatric transport team managers. *Pediatr Emerg Care* 2001;**17**:22–7.

Drugs

Mildenhall LFJ, Pavuluri NN, Bowman ED. Safety of synthetic surfactant use before preterm newborn transport. *J Pediatr Child Health* 1999;**35**:530–5.

Royal College of Paediatrics and Child Health. *Medicines for Children*. London: RCPCH Publications, 1999.

Shann F. *Drug Doses*, 11th edn. Melbourne: Collective Pty, 2001.

Index